Headache

WHAT DO I DO NOW?

What Do I Do Now? – Pain Medicine

SERIES EDITORS

Mark P Jensen and Lynn R. Webster

PUBLISHED AND FORTHCOMING TITLES:

Headache

Edited by
Olivia Begasse de Dhaem, MD, FAHS
Assistant Professor of Neurology
Department of Neurology, University of Connecticut
Hartford HealthCare
Milford, CT, USA

Carolyn Bernstein, MD, FAHS
Assistant Professor of Neurology
Lavine Family Distinguished Chair, Neurology
Harvard Medical School
Boston, MA, USA

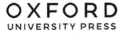

OXFORD
UNIVERSITY PRESS

OXFORD
UNIVERSITY PRESS

Oxford University Press is a department of the University of Oxford. It furthers
the University's objective of excellence in research, scholarship, and education
by publishing worldwide. Oxford is a registered trade mark of Oxford University
Press in the UK and certain other countries.

Published in the United States of America by Oxford University Press
198 Madison Avenue, New York, NY 10016, United States of America.

Library of Congress Cataloging-in-Publication Data
Names: Begasse de Dhaem, Olivia, editor. | Bernstein, Carolyn, editor.
Title: Headache / edited by Olivia Begasse de Dhaem and Carolyn Bernstein.
Other titles: Headache (Begasse de Dhaem)
Description: New York, NY : Oxford University Press, [2023] |
Includes bibliographical references and index. |
Identifiers: LCCN 2022040726 (print) | LCCN 2022040727 (ebook) |
ISBN 9780197659441 (paperback) | ISBN 9780197659465 (epub) | ISBN 9780197659472
Subjects: MESH: Headache—etiology | Headache—diagnosis |
Diagnosis, Differential. | Headache—therapy
Classification: LCC RC392 (print) | LCC RC392 (ebook) | NLM WL 342 |
DDC 616.8/4913—dc23/eng/20221128
LC record available at https://lccn.loc.gov/2022040726
LC ebook record available at https://lccn.loc.gov/2022040727

DOI: 10.1093/med/9780197659441.001.0001

Printed by Marquis Book Printing, Canada

This book is dedicated to:

Hadi, Lila, my parents, Nicolas, Broca, Oscar, Max, Firmin, Père. I am eternally grateful to them for all their love and support.

Dr. Carolyn A. Bernstein, who has been a generous and inspiring mentor, friend, life coach, and co-editor.

My mentors who have significantly contributed to my development: Drs. Christophe Schmit, Gerard F. Iwantsch, Cris Poor, James A. Ciaccio, Bob Brodner, Bill (William C.) Turner, Norma Braun, Anil K. Lalwani, Mia T. Minen, Carolyn B. Britton, Linda D. Lewis, Jay P. Mohr, Jinsy A. Andrews, Phil Muskin, David Dodick, Denise Chou, Elizabeth W. Loder, Robert E. Shapiro, Paul B. Rizzoli, Thomas N. Ward, Rebecca C. Burch, Bill (William Joseph) Mullally, Louise Resor, Brian E. McGeeney.

—Olivia Begasse de Dhaem, MD, FAHS

I would like to dedicate this book to all the wonderful patients who have taught me so much about headache, and my amazing collaborator and co-editor Olivia Begasse de Dhaem, MD.

—Carolyn Bernstein, MD, FAHS
Lavine Family Distinguished Chair in Neurology

Contents

Preface

A lot has changed in the field of headache medicine recently with the ever-changing understanding of the pathophysiology of headache disorders and the development of new medications developed specifically for migraine. However, the main principles and reasons to get involved in the field of headache medicine remain. A lot can be done by being present, supportive, and listening to patients with empathy, admiration for their courage, and open-mindedness. Headache diseases are mostly diagnosed with clinical history. Open-ended questions and a thorough history are crucial to make the correct diagnosis. When in doubt, it is never wrong to schedule a quick follow-up appointment to monitor the patient closely and get more information. Although the diagnosis of primary headache disorders relies on clinical history, an astute neurological examination with special consideration for the cranial nerves is required to screen for secondary etiologies. There is no way to predict what treatment will work best for patients, and some patience and trial and error are needed when developing and optimizing the treatment plan. Everyone is unique and benefits from a unique, personalized treatment. Decision-making should be shared between patients and providers as a team. Patient education is crucial to empower them and help them in their management of the disease. Multimodal approaches with medications, devices, behavioral therapies, and complementary and integrative medicine therapies are synergistic. Comorbidities must be evaluated and addressed. Headache medicine is such a rewarding field because a lot can be done for patients. These core principles persist through time and make the beauty of our field. The field changes so fast, there may be some changes between book editions, but we do not expect them to significantly alter the teaching from our book.

This book was written as a practical case-based, easy-to-read resource for all clinicians, providers, and trainees who take care of patients with headache disorders.

Contributors

Ashley Alex, MD
Clinical Assistant Professor
Department of Neurology
Jacobs School of Medicine and
Biomedical Sciences
State University of New York
Buffalo, NY, USA

**Olivia Begasse de Dhaem,
MD, FAHS**
Assistant Professor of Neurology
Department of Neurology
University of Connecticut
Hartford HealthCare
Milford, CT, USA

Carolyn Bernstein, MD, FAHS
Assistant Professor of Neurology
Lavine Family Distinguished Chair,
Neurology
Harvard Medical School
Boston, MA, USA

Bryce Buchowicz, MD
Assistant Professor of
Neuro-ophthalmology
Department of Ophthalmology
University of Florida College of
Medicine
Gainesville, FL, USA

Ian Carroll, MD, MS
Department of Anesthesiology
Perioperative and Pain Medicine
Stanford University
Stanford, CA, USA

Claire E. J. Ceriani, MD
Assistant Professor
Department of Neurology
Jefferson Headache Center
Thomas Jefferson University
Hospital
Philadelphia, PA, USA

Chia-Chun Chiang, MD
Assistant Professor of Neurology
Department of Neurology
Mayo Clinic
Rochester, MN, USA

Jessica Gautreaux, MD
Associate Professor
Department of Neurology
Louisiana State University Health
Sciences Center
New Orleans, LA, USA

**Mohammad Hadi Gharedaghi,
MD, MPH**
Anesthesiology Attending
Department of Anesthesia
Stamford Hospital
Stamford, CT, USA

Ashley Parham Ghiaseddin, MD
Clinical Associate Professor
Department of Neurosurgery
University of Florida College of
Medicine
Gainesville, FL, USA

Elena Haight, BS
Geisel School of Medicine at
Dartmouth
Hanover, NH, USA

**Carly E. Harrington,
AGPCNP-BC, RN**
Adult Nurse Practitioner
Department of Neurology
Dent Neurologic Institute
Amherst, NY, USA

**María F. Hernández-Nuño de la
Rosa, DDS, MS**
Assistant Professor and Director of
Clinical Research
Department of Oral and
Maxillofacial Surgery
Tufts School of Dental
Medicine
Boston, MA, USA

**Julie H. Huang-Lionnet,
MD, MPH**
Executive Medical Director
Interventional Pain Medicine
Greenwich Health
Greenwich, CT, USA

Shivang Joshi, MD, MPH, RPh
Associate Adjunct Professor
University of Buffalo School of
Pharmacy
Dent Neurologic Institute
Amherst, NY, USA

Eric A. Kaiser, MD, PhD
Assistant Professor
Department of Neurology
University of Pennsylvania
Philadelphia, PA, USA

Saad Kanaan, MD
Assistant Professor of Neurology
Department of Neurology &
Rehabilitation Medicine
University of Cincinnati
Cincinnati, OH, USA

Deena E. Kuruvilla, MD, FAHS
Medical Director
Westport Headache Institute
Westport, CT, USA

Sandhya Mehla, MD
Assistant Professor
Department of Neurology
University of Connecticut School
of Medicine
Farmington, CT, USA
Headache Specialist
Vascular Neurologist
Hartford Healthcare
Headache Center
Ayer Neuroscience Institute
Norwich, CT, USA

Kaitlyn Melnick, MD
Resident Physician
Department of Neurosurgery
University of Florida College of
Medicine
Gainesville, FL, USA

Natalia Murinova, MD, MHA, FAAN
Clinical Associate Professor
Department of Neurology
Director of the Neurology
Headache Clinic
University of Washington
Seattle, WA, USA

Yulia Orlova, MD
Assistant Professor
Department of Neurology
University of Florida College of
Medicine
Gainesville, FL, USA

Bridget LaMonica Ostrem, MD, PhD
Instructor
Department of Neurology
Brigham and Women's Hospital,
Massachusetts General Hospital
Boston, MA, USA

Carrie E. Robertson, MD, FAHS
Assistant Professor
Department of Neurology
Mayo Clinic College of Medicine
Rochester, MN, USA

Huma U. Sheikh, MD
CEO
NY Neurology Medicine, PC
New York, NY, USA
Assistant Professor
Department of Neurology
Icahn-Mount Sinai School of
Medicine
New York, NY, USA

Victor C. Wang, MD
Instructor
Department of Neurology
Brigham and Women's Hospital,
Harvard Medical School
Boston, MA, USA

Hsiangkuo Yuan, MD, PhD
Associate Professor
Department of Neurology
Jefferson Headache Center,
Thomas Jefferson University
Hospital
Philadelphia, PA, USA

1 Clinical Pearls and Red Flags

**Carolyn Bernstein and
Olivia Begasse de Dhaem**

INTRODUCTION

Headache is one of the most challenging and common presentations in a clinical office visit, the emergency department, or an inpatient room. The word "headache" means different things to different patients, and it is up to you to figure out if something serious is occurring, to look for "red flag" emergency signs, and to start a treatment plan.

HISTORY AND EXAMINATION

Taking a good history is crucial, especially in headache medicine, because most of our diagnoses rely on symptoms. We suggest letting the patient describe what they are experiencing uninterrupted first. Often, you'll get plenty of information that will help to guide your approach. Listening to your patient without interruption first will also help build trust and might save you time in the long run.

Establishing early on whether the headache is "new" and/or "different" from prior headaches, the "first" or "worst" headache of life is critical. Here are the basic questions of a headache history that will help narrow your differential:

1. When did the problem start?
2. Have you ever experienced it before?
3. Where is the pain located?
4. What is the quality of the pain (e.g. stabbing, pressing, pounding, throbbing)?
5. Is it continuous? If not, how long does the pain last?
6. Have you taken any medication or tried any treatment for it?
7. Are you nauseated? Have you vomited?
8. Do sound or light bother you?
9. Do your eyes tear? Does your nose run? Do you have sweating in your face?
10. Any recent trauma?
11. Any recent travel?
12. Has anyone been sick at home?
13. (Current question) Did you have COVID 19?
14. Do you feel better lying down or standing?

15. Are you weak in an arm or a leg?
16. Any blurred vision? Double vision?
17. Are you dizzy or spinning?
18. Do you have a family history of headache?

It is also important to ask patients what their biggest concern is and what their expectations are from the current visit, to ensure you are working with them as a team. Once you have a differential diagnosis in your mind, especially for patients with a long history of headaches, it is helpful to ask more questions to assess comorbidities and headache-related disability. For example, ask about trauma, abuse, stressors, mood disorders, sleep, hydration, and other pain disorders. To evaluate for disability, you can ask how different their lives would be if they did not have headaches.

Second, a neurologic exam should be performed with funduscopic evaluation and thorough cranial nerve examination, as well as deep tendon reflexes and other basic components.

FLAGS

The first goal in the evaluation of a headache is to assess whether the headache is primary or secondary. Primary headaches occur independently without a pathological etiology. Secondary headaches occur as the result of an underlying cause such as disease or trauma. Secondary headaches affect about 18% of people with a headache. Differentiating between the two will guide evaluation, management, and prognosis. Sometimes it is impossible to clinically differentiate between primary and secondary headaches and further work-up is needed. The different flags might guide your decisions to pursue further work-up.

Red flags should alert you that action needs to take place immediately, such as imaging or lumbar puncture. Orange flags are alarming if accompanied by other red or orange flags. The SNNOOP10 mnemonic makes it easier to remember the red flags: (1) **S**ystemic symptoms including fever, (2) **N**eoplasm, (3) **N**eurologic deficit, (4) abrupt or sudden **O**nset, (5) **O**lder than 50 years of age, (6) recent change in **P**attern, (7) **P**ositional headache,(8) **P**recipitated by sneezing, coughing, exercise, (9) **P**apilledema on fundoscopic exam, (10) **P**regnancy, (11) **P**ainful eye with autonomic features, (12) **P**rogressive headache, (13) **P**ost-traumatic onset, (14) immunosuppressive **P**athology, (15) frequent or new **P**ainkiller use.

There is a new mnemonic, SAIL, for red flags that warrant both brain MRI and head and neck vessel imaging in patients with aura: (1) **S**ide-locked aura, (2) **A**typical aura, (3) **I**ncreasing aura frequency, or (4) **L**ate onset of aura.

Here are some tips for next steps in the evaluation once you encounter red flags:

- Fever with a new headache should prompt concerns for meningitis, especially in people who are immune compromised. Do not be fooled by lack of nuchal rigidity.
- Obtain a non-contrast head CT if there is any concern for bleeding, such as anticoagulation use or patient who has sustained trauma. Loss of consciousness with head trauma followed by an alert period can portend an epidural headache.
- Try to get a brain MRI rapidly for a new or different headache in a patient over age 50, for focal neurologic signs on examination such as hemi-body weakness, and for post-traumatic headaches. If the patient describes a positional headache, MRI is the study of choice, potentially followed by a lumbar puncture to assess pressure. Tumor headaches are often more slowly intensifying, but not always. Patients may hemorrhage into a mass, or develop severe edema around the lesion, which can cause vomiting and altered level of consciousness. Again, if the headache is new or worsening, imaging is key, and MRI brain is preferred unless there is a concern for acute blood.
- Unilateral temple pain (or bilateral) in a person over age 50 should trigger an evaluation for giant cell arteritis (GCA). Check ESR and CRP, and either biopsy or perform a precision temporal artery ultrasound. If you are concerned about GCA, do not wait for biopsy results before starting steroids.

Although the presence of green flags is suggestive of a primary headache disorder, you need to look for red and orange flags and evaluate as needed if one red flag and/or several orange flags are present. The proposed green flags include (1) the current headache having started during childhood, (2) temporal relationship between the headache and menstrual cycles, (3) the presence of headache-free days, and (4) headache similarity with close family members. Be careful; a long history of a primary headache disorder is not always reassuring. For example, migraine is associated with a higher risk of postpartum stroke, cerebral sinus venous thrombosis, and reversible cerebral vasoconstrictive syndrome.

CLINICAL PEARLS

Here are a few pieces of wisdom that will help manage your patients' pain and symptoms:

- Have your patient keep a detailed calendar of headache frequency, symptoms, and acute medications used. You will obtain useful insight into questions about medication adaptation headache, for example.
- Use the visual aura rating scale to screen for aura. Most patients with aura have visual aura at some point.
- Review risk factors for migraine chronification with patients who have episodic migraine as part of prevention efforts.
- Listen to your patients. Show respect. Be supportive. Provide them with different therapeutic options and education.
- Once you are certain that the patient has a primary headache and that red flags have been ruled out, anti-inflammatories such as IM or IV ketorolac can help tremendously in the acute setting.
- Consider a quick six-day steroid taper for status migrainosus unless contra-indicated.
- Pure menstrual migraine can often be managed by suppressing hormonal cycling; be sure your patient does not have aura. Given the increased risk of stroke in people with migraine with aura, we recommend avoiding exogenous estrogen. If OCP is safe to use, try continuous dosing.

CONCLUSION

This chapter is meant to provide general tips for the evaluation of headache disorders. Chapters in this book will guide you more specifically through approaches to different types of headaches. If you remember two things from this chapter: (1) take a good history and (2) figure out whether the headache is new and/or different.

Further Reading

1. Do TP, Remmers A, Schytz HW, et al. "Red and orange flags for secondary headaches in clinical practice: SNNOOP10 list." *Neurology.* 2019;92(3):134–144. https://doi.org/10.1212/WNL.0000000000006697
2. Pohl H, Do TP, García-Azorín D, et al. "Green flags and headache: A concept study using the Delphi method." *Headache.* 2021;61(2):300–309. doi:10.1111/head.14054
3. Evans RW, Burch RC, Frishberg BM, et al. "Neuroimaging for migraine: The American Headache Society systematic review and evidence-based guideline." *Headache.* 2020;60(2):318–336. https://doi.org/10.1111/head.13720
4. Eriksen MK, Thomsen LL, Olesen J. "The Visual Aura Rating Scale (VARS) for migraine aura diagnosis." *Cephalalgia.* 2005;25(10):801–810. https://doi.org/10.1111/j.1468-2982.2005.00955.x
5. Scher AI, Midgette LA, Lipton RB. "Risk factors for headache chronification." *Headache.* 2008;48(1):16–25. https://doi.org/10.1111/j.1526-4610.2007.00970.x
6. Thomsen AV, et al. "Symptomatic migraine: a systematic review to establish a clinically important diagnostic entity." *Headache.* 2021; https://doi.org/10.1111/head.14187

2 Telemedicine for Headache: Welcome to the Virtual World

Carolyn Bernstein and

Olivia Begasse de Dhaem

The COVID 19 pandemic has moved us all to unique places in our practice of medicine, including virtual patient care. Medical care delivery will be forever different as a result. A review of "best virtual practice" is in order.

Connecting with a patient via a virtual portal is a brave new world. You, as medical provider, need to pull on multiple areas of your own brain activation. You are looking at your patient simultaneously as you look at the medical record, imaging studies, your own notes in progress, and whatever else pops onto your screen despite your best efforts to turn everything else off. You need a quiet, private place to conduct these visits, and it may be difficult if you are working from somewhere other than the office.

The fewer personal effects in your own background the better. We have all seen special effects so that you can appear to be standing on a beach, or in front of the Golden Gate Bridge. This is distracting and confusing for your patient, who is likely seeing a larger image of you than vice versa. In addition, the false backgrounds have some odd effects so that if you lean back or turn your head, part of you may disappear. An empty space is often best, calming for the patient and less distracting. If you don't have a plain white wall, it may be worth investing in a simple screen that you can place behind your workspace. And remember to make things as ergonomically comfortable as you can. A low keyboard, a good chair, adequate lighting, and fast internet will make the visit easier for both you and the patient.

Establishing a connection and trust with the patient can be harder in a virtual setting. Give patients time to talk uninterrupted. When you talk, make pauses to enable patients to process the information and ask any questions that may arise. Use positive body language. Make sure to look at the camera to appear to be making eye contact. It is helpful to place the view of the patient on your screen so that it is as close as possible to your camera, so it is easier for you to maintain virtual eye contact. Acknowledge the limitations of virtual visits and establish a clear follow-up plan to show patients you are there for them.

Creating a template for your notes is also helpful and will remind you to check the patient's birthdate (for security), remind them that the visit is not being recorded, is encrypted, and is not a substitute for a live visit. It will also help you move through key elements of a headache evaluation so that if there are background distractions, you won't lose your thought process. Once you move through the history and background details, you can do a fairly thorough virtual neurologic exam. It's very helpful if there is someone else at the patient's home that you can guide through some simple sensory and strength testing. But if not, you can still perform the exam, excluding funduscopic exam and pupillary responses (although you can look for asymmetry) and reflexes. Have the patient draw their fingers down their face to check light touch symmetry. Ask them to stroke each arm and check for pronator drift and finger to nose. They can do a squat unassisted, which gives you a sense of lower body strength. Heel/toe/tandem are all components to evaluate as well as Romberg test. You want to be sure to emphasize that the patient should not do anything if they feel they may fall, as you are not able to catch them.

Once history and exam are complete, we recommend discussing the diagnosis and starting the treatment plan, being certain to share exactly what you are including in the note with the patient. Often, reading them your assessment and plan, and documenting that you did so, can reinforce your suggestions. You can also copy-paste your assessment and plan, spell any complicated words or the diagnosis, or write down key information in the chat. With the Cures Act now in effect, it is even more important to ensure that patients understand precisely what your formulation is and what their treatment will entail. Also, document the follow-up plan carefully.

Many patients enjoy the convenience of virtual visits. They don't have to drive to an appointment, miss work, arrange childcare, and pay for parking. There is, however, some laxity that has increased over time. Patients may try to conduct the visit while driving or in a moving car. They may have family or co-workers present or may be in a vacation location that might prohibit a telemedicine visit. We recommend having staff pre-screen patients and review visit etiquette. You can always reschedule the visit if the conditions are suboptimal or unsafe, such as the patient driving.

Telemedicine discriminates against our patients who don't have tech access or who are unable to understand how to use it. Some patients also do not have the option of finding a quiet and safe space without distractions at home. Live options should always be available, and patients should be respected if they select to be seen in person.

While we are all eager to move forward from the pandemic, telehealth will be here to stay in some form going forward. These tips may help you to navigate more easily between virtual and live.

Further Reading

1. Begasse de Dhaem O, Bernstein C. "Headache virtual visit toolbox: The transition from bedside manners to webside manners." *Headache.* 2020;60(8):1743–1746. https://doi.org/10.1111/head.13885
2. Klein BC, Busis NA. "COVID-19 is catalyzing the adoption of teleneurology." *Neurology.* 2020;94(21):903–904. https://doi.org/10.1212/WNL.0000000000009494
3. Govindarajan R, Anderson ER, Hesselbrock RR, et al. "Developing an outline for teleneurology curriculum. AAN Telemedicine Work Group recommendations." *Neurology.* 2017;89(9):951–959. https://doi.org/10.1212/WNL.0000000000004285
4. Hatcher-Martin JM, Busis NA, Cohen BH, et al. "American Academy of Neurology telehealth position statement." *Neurology.* 2021;97(7):334–339. https://doi.org/10.1212/WNL.0000000000012185

3 The Answer Is Not Always a Medicine

Carolyn Bernstein

KJ is a 35-year-old woman with migraine meeting the International Classification of Headache Disorders 3rd edition (ICHD-3) criteria for migraine. She has 2–4 migraine attacks per month with neck pain, unilateral throbbing, and photophobia. There is no associated aura, no focal numbness or weakness, and no vertigo. After the acute attack, she reports 24 hours of fatigue that impacts her work ability. She is adamant that she prefers not to take medication nor use any devices if possible. She spends her days at a desk job with little activity. She snacks on processed foods at irregular times, drinks little water, and tells you that she feels very stressed. She has seen other clinicians for her headaches but didn't like the offers of prescription acute and preventive medications or devices. She is sexually active with a partner with sperm and does not use contraception. Her sleep is poor as well. She is hoping that you will recommend non-pharma complementary and integrative therapies.

What do I do now?

Evaluation

The work-up for this patient would be identical to any other patient with likely migraine. A careful history, diary details if possible, a thorough neurologic exam, and a review of old records are all essential. She has had identical events beginning at age 18, occurring several times a month, not associated with her menstrual period. Her exam is normal, there are no flags, and imaging and other investigations are not warranted. She has migraine without aura meeting ICHD-3 criteria.

Education

It is helpful for both the patient and the clinician to have an open conversation on what the patient's goals and expectations are around treatment. It is also important to explain the different options that can be offered to the patient. Medications do exist, both for acute treatment and preventive, that are well-evidenced with newer biologics offering potential treatments with fewer side effects. KJ is adamant that she does not want to try any medication nor devices. The decision about including complementary and integrative medicine (CIM) is never binary, however. Patients should be encouraged to choose the treatment plan that is best for them in particular—true "personalized medicine."

It can be helpful to divide CIM therapies into touch therapies, movement therapies, mindfulness therapies, and coaching/lifestyle interventions including herbs/vitamins. Touch therapies include chiropractic work, craniosacral therapy, massage, and acupuncture. Tai Chi, yoga with a focus on restorative therapies, Feldenkreis work (structural and gait postures and movement focus), and exercise can all be considered as movement therapies when used as treatments. Mindfulness therapies can be divided into cognitive behavioral therapy (CBT), meditation focused practices, and third-line therapies such as acceptance and commitment therapies. Finally, the integrative coaching therapies are focused on helping patients to make small and meaningful changes in their lives via wellness, nutrition, or other lifestyle changes. Functional medicine specialists can provide informed data around the use of herbs and vitamins. It is critical to remember that these supplements can have side effects and should be approached with knowledge and caution. It is important to review those safe in pregnancy (since the patient is not using contraception). We encourage readers to try

TABLE 3.1 Recipe for a day of complete nutritious plant-based migraine-friendly diet with higher omega-3 and lower omega-6 fats

Breakfast	· 1 cup oatmeal + 1/2 cup fresh or frozen berries · Green tea
Snack	· 5 walnuts or Brazil nuts

Lunch	· Happy big bowl:
	  - 1/2 cup steamed broccolis (you can buy organic broccoli florets ready to heat in the microwave)
	  - 1 handful of watercress
	  - 1/2 avocado
	  - 3 minced scallions
	  - 1/2 cup black beans (canned and rinsed)
	  - 1/2 cup buckwheat
	  - 1 tablespoon flaxseed on the top
	· Dressing:
	  - 1 tablespoon of lemon juice
	  - 1/4 cup unsweetened nut-milk
	  - 1/4 teaspoon turmeric
	  - 1 teaspoon ginger powder
	  - 1 clove of minced garlic
	· Dessert: 1 portion of watermelon

Snack	· Fresh red grapes with seeds and skin

Dinner	· Whole wheat pasta
	· Red sauce:
	  - 1 tablespoon of plant cold-pressed oil
	  - 2 peeled and cut red onions
	  - 1 bunch peeled and cut organic carrot
	  - 2 stalks of celery, cut and peeled
	  - Place in a plan, close the lid, cook at low heat for 30 minutes, then add 3 cut red tomatoes, cayenne pepper, oregano, and thyme
	  - Keep it at low heat for another 15 minutes then blend together.
	  - Add 1 cup of drained rinsed beans to the sauce.
	· Dessert: 1 portion pineapple

Tips	· You can cook the whole packages of oatmeal, buckwheat, beans and keep them refrigerated and reheat as needed during the week

—Courtesy of Karine Dehogne, AFPA-certified Holistic Nutritionist some of these CIM therapies such as acupuncture or craniosacral therapy themselves. Treatments can be focused on a variety of conditions including headaches. Cardiac coherent breathing is a simple technique of taking six slow breaths per minute, in for five counts and out for five counts. It has been shown to decrease anxiety and calm the sympathetic nervous system.

Management

KJ is excited to participate in shared decision-making with her clinician. A plan that includes integrative health coaching to work on improved sleep, hydration, and exercise is very successful. Integrative nutrition focuses on small changes in her food consumption including regular small meals with complex carbohydrates, primarily plant-based. Table 3.1 provides an example of a healthy migraine-friendly diet. It is important to make dietary changes progressively and to eat foods that make you happy and feel good. A healthy diet is good if it is sustainable and makes you happy in the long run. A course of acupuncture decreases the frequency of KJ's headaches. She begins to develop her own yoga practice with assistance from an individualized yoga teacher. She is satisfied with this plan and appreciates the holistic lifestyle approach, and although she continues to have occasional migraine attacks, they are less frequent and easier to manage. In addition, she has embraced the autonomy of her health decisions and feels empowered, which has positive effects in the rest of her life.

CIM approaches can also complement pharmacological treatment. They are not exclusive and can be synergic.

KEY POINTS TO REMEMBER

- Correct diagnosis and evaluation are key
- Shared decision-making around treatment is beneficial for both clinician and patients
- Familiarize yourself with CIM therapies, experientially if possible
- Build a base of CIM practitioners that you trust
- Continue to evaluate outcomes carefully
- Make sure that treatments are safe and that practitioners are licensed and experienced

Further Reading

1. Millstine D, Chen CY, Bauer B. "Complementary and integrative medicine in the management of headache." *BMJ.* 2017;357:j1805. https://doi.org/10.1136/bmj.j1805
2. Wells R, Baute V, Wahbeh H. "Complementary and integrative medicine for neurologic conditions." *Med Clin North Am.* 2017;101(5):881–893. https://doi.org/10.1016/j.mcna.2017.04.006
3. Wells RE, Buethin J, Granetzke L. "Complementary and integrative medicine for episodic migraine: an update of evidence from the last 3 years." *Curr Pain Headache Rep.* 2019;23(2):10. https://doi.org/10.1007/s11916-019-0750-8

4 I'm So Anxious About My Headache that I Can't Breathe

Carolyn Bernstein

Joe is a 40-year-old man and lives with his husband and two children ages 4 and 8. He works in venture capital and is the chief earner for the family (his husband stays home with the children). Work pressures have been increasing, and there are ongoing financial worries. Joe has not been a "headache person" and has generally been well. He was a college athlete, playing soccer, but his activity level has decreased since having children and he rarely exercises. He comes to see you describing a new generalized headache without any specific features. He denies photo and phonophobia as well as nausea. There are no visual changes, and the headache is not positional. He denies weakness and numbness. The pain is aching, and if he is distracted he does not notice it. It is worse at night or when he is in a stressful work situation. He describes feeling overwhelmed and is frightened that he may have a brain tumor or other lesion that is causing his headache.

What do I do now?

Diagnosis

Careful history-taking cues you to a pattern of anxiety-triggered headaches. Detailed neurologic exam is entirely normal. Joe's husband has accompanied him, and with permission you are able to discern concerns for situational anxiety about illness, mortality, finances, and child care. Joe did not have a history of anxiety, although in retrospect there were previous indicators that had been ignored. MRI brain is completely normal (expected, but necessary for this patient to move past the fear that he had a brain tumor). He agrees to a psychiatric evaluation, and a diagnosis of generalized anxiety disorder (GAD) is made. The patient also begins to keep a diary, and it is clear that the headache presents when his anxiety increases. You are able to make a diagnosis of secondary headache: headache attributed to GAD, a diagnosis present in the appendix of the International Classification of Headache Disorders 3rd edition (A12.8). You reassure the patient that this is totally treatable.

Education

Patients like this warrant a thoughtful evaluation, as people with anxiety can certainly have other headache etiologies. Imaging is appropriate if the patient's anxiety is such that they are unable to function without concrete reassurance via imaging. Before ordering any imaging, though, it is important to discuss with the patients common incidental findings, such as small white matter changes or pituitary microadenomas that may be found, so that they don't panic if somehow the MRI report gets to them before you call them. It is important to be certain that the patient is fully vested in ongoing counseling, as the headache is unlikely to otherwise resolve. Patients value an explanation of how stress can trigger or worsen pain, and that you expect a significant improvement once the anxiety is addressed. A gross description of brain anatomy with the shared pathways between anxiety, insomnia, and headache may help validate patients' symptoms and empower them. The key point is to recognize and clarify anxiety as a trigger. Patients should not be incorrectly diagnosed with migraine or other primary headache disorder, for example.

Anxiety has profound effects on immune function and inflammation. It can be crippling for patients caught in an anxiety attack—and may be more recognizable if there are signs of acute sympathetic hyperactivity such as tachycardia and elevated blood pressure—but bouts of anxiety may present differently, and headache can be triggered by anxiety. Other somatic symptoms may present as well, such as gastrointestinal symptoms, body pain, or fatigue. A careful review of systems will help you to clarify the diagnosis, and having psychiatric colleagues to whom you can refer is essential.

Management

Once diagnosis is made, the next question is how to treat. Patients may feel that they need to "tough it out" and conquer the anxiety unaided. Both medication and complementary and integrative medicine (CIM) therapies have a role for these patients. CIM therapies are further discussed in Chapter 3, "The Answer Is Not Always a Medicine." SSRIs can be tremendously helpful for anxiety and for the anticipation of the next headache; careful titration is essential. Beta blockers will help with the autonomic nervous system component of the anxiety, which may help to resolve the headache. It is always important to promote therapy, whether talk therapy or a biobehavioral technique such as cognitive behavioral therapy (CBT) or Eye Movement Desensitization and Reprocessing (EMDR), which patients can use when they feel the anxiety ramping up. Before referring patients to CBT or other therapies, it is important to discuss what these therapies entail to ensure patients know what to expect. Joe would likely benefit from re-engaging in an exercise program and trying some sort of mindfulness practice.

It is important to assess how much acute medication (if any) the patient is using, as medication adaptation headache may be triggered in addition to the headache secondary to anxiety. While an NSAID may be helpful in the moment, it is important to treat the etiology of the headache and to work on managing the anxiety. Be certain to reassure the patient that you will not abandon them and will continue to work together to manage the headache, but also to stress that the psychiatric treatment is equally important. By removing the stigma, understanding the etiology, and creating a care plan that synchs with the patient's wishes, you will help to resolve this challenging headache.

Further Reading

1. Pérez-Muñoz A, et al. "Behavioral interventions for migraine." *Neurol Clin.* 2019;37(4):789–813. https://doi.org/10.1016/j.ncl.2019.07.003
2. Minen, MT, et al. "Migraine and its psychiatric comorbidities." *J Neurol Neurosurg Psychiatry.* 2016;87(7):741–749. https://doi.org/10.1136/jnnp-2015-312233

5 Pregnancy Pearls

Olivia Begasse de Dhaem and
Carolyn Bernstein

PLANNING PRIOR TO PREGNANCY

- Reassurance about likely course. Unfortunately, about 20% of women avoid pregnancy out of fear of pregnancy complications related to migraine, migraine worsening in pregnancy, and medications hurting the fetus. However, most women see a significant improvement in their migraine attacks during pregnancy. During the first trimester, about 50% of women see an improvement, and 8% notice a worsening in their headaches. By the third trimester, 87% of women have an improvement in their migraine attacks.
- Folic acid supplementation will not affect headaches, but it is important to discuss it in case this has not yet been explained to the patient by anyone.
- Wean off/stop medications that are not safe in pregnancy (topiramate, valproic acid, venlafaxine, ACEi, ARB, CGRP monoclonal antibodies). Due to their long half-lives, it is recommended that CGRP monoclonal antibodies are stopped 6 months before conception. Discuss other treatment options that are relatively safer in pregnancy.

HEADACHE IN PREGNANCY

- More than half of new-onset headaches in pregnancy are secondary. It is important to obtain a careful history, vitals (especially blood pressure), and a thorough neurological examination looking for focal abnormalities. There should be a low threshold for further work-up. Key questions to ask include:
  - Is the headache new?
  - Any neurological symptoms such as confusion, blurry vision, or seizures?
  - What is the phenotype of the headache? How acute was the onset of the pain? Did it reach maximal peak of intensity upon its start (thunderclap)? How long does the headache last? How long has this been going on?

- Any family history of headache?
- What is the stage of the pregnancy?
- What medications are you taking?
- Have you had any pregnancy complications so far?
- Have you had nausea? Difficulty eating? Assess for poor nutrition.
- How has your sleep been? Lack of sleep will contribute to headaches.
- How has your mood been? Do you feel anxious, sad, depressed?
- The differential for new headache or a change of headache in pregnancy includes:
  - Hypertensive disorders such as preeclampsia, eclampsia, posterior reversible encephalopathy syndrome, HELLP syndrome (hemolysis, elevated liver enzymes, low platelet count), arterial hypertension, reversible cerebral vasoconstrictive syndrome.
  - Cerebral sinus venous thrombosis, infection, pituitary apoplexy, intracranial bleed, idiopathic intracranial hypertension.

MIGRAINE IN PREGNANCY

- Although 80% of headaches in pregnancy are migraine in women with a prior headache history, it is crucial to rule out secondary etiologies, as migraine is also a risk factor for pregnancy complications such as gestational hypertension, preeclampsia, pulmonary embolism, stroke, and myocardial infarction. Migraine treatment does not reduce the migraine-related increased risk of those complications.
- Acute treatment considerations
  - The first line is acetaminophen with or without metoclopramide.
  - The second line is sumatriptan.
  - Cyclobenzaprine, lidocaine nasal spray, and use of the transcutaneous supraorbital nerve stimulator can be considered.
  - Acute treatments to be avoided in pregnancy include NSAIDs in the first and third trimesters due to increased risk of miscarriage and premature closure of the ductus arteriosus;, gepants and ditans (due to current lack of data in pregnancy); opioids (not

recommended as migraine acute treatments); and butalbital-containing compounds such as fioricet (due to increased risk of fetal heart defects and withdrawal seizures).
- Preventive treatment considerations
  - Preventive medication options include cyproheptadine, memantine, propranolol, verapamil, regular nerve blocks with lidocaine (no bupivacaine, no steroids).
  - Non-pharmacological preventive treatments include riboflavin, enzyme CoQ10, cognitive behavioral therapy, progressive muscle relaxation, biofeedback, regular physical exercise.
  - Again, topiramate, valproic acid, venlafaxine, ACEi, ARB, and CGRP monoclonal antibodies should be avoided.

POST-PARTUM HEADACHE

- A careful evaluation and possibly further work-up are necessary to rule out secondary causes such as stroke, intracranial bleed, embolic infarct due to amniotic fluid, cerebral sinus venous thrombosis, reversible cerebral vasoconstrictive syndrome, pre-eclampsia, eclampsia, Sheehan's syndrome, cervicocephalic artery dissection.
- About 1.5% of epidurals are followed by a post–dural puncture headache. The first-line management is bed rest, hydration, and caffeine, but an epidural blood patch may be necessary.
- Although the threshold for work-up should be low, and post-partum headaches have to be taken seriously, it is reassuring to know that the most common cause of post-partum headache is the resurgence of a prior primary headache disorder.
- Breastfeeding delays the resurgence of migraine attacks.

MIGRAINE AND LACTATION

- Acute treatment considerations:
  - The first-line options are acetaminophen, ibuprofen.
  - The second-line options are ondansetron and diclofenac.

- The third-line options are eletriptan (the triptan with the lowest breast milk concentration), sumatriptan, rizatriptan.
- Domperidone can help with both the headache/nausea and breast milk production.
- Butalbital-containing agents should be avoided, as they are not recommended as acute migraine treatments and they can cause infant sedation.
- Preventive treatment considerations:
  - First-line options include verapamil, propranolol.
  - Second-line options include amitriptyline, nortriptyline, memantine.
  - Riboflavin is considered safe. Women should be informed it will tint their breast milk yellow.
  - To date, there are no data on the safety of OnabotulinumtoxinA in breastfeeding.

KEY POINTS TO REMEMBER

- Migraine improves for most women in pregnancy. Breastfeeding usually delays the recurrence of migraine attacks.
- Headaches in pregnancy and in the post-partum period should be thoroughly evaluated due to the high risk of a secondary etiology.
- It is important to reassure women that there are treatment options for headache in pregnancy and during the breastfeeding period.

Further Reading
1. Burch R. "Headache in pregnancy and the puerperium." *Neurol Clin.* 2019;37(1):31–51. https://doi.org/10.1016/j.ncl.2018.09.004
2. Pavlović JM. "Headache in women." *Continuum.* 2021;27(3):686–702. https://doi.org/10.1212/CON.0000000000001010
3. Saldanha IJ, et al. "Management of primary headaches during pregnancy, postpartum, and breastfeeding: A systematic review." *Headache.* 2021;61(1):11–43. https://doi.org/10.1111/head.14041

6 "Why Do I Have So Many Headaches?"

Natalia Murinova

A 27-year-old woman is having an average of 16 headache days per month. Headaches became a problem 2 years ago. The average pain severity is 7/10. The most severe headaches are rated 9/10. The headaches often last more than 4 hours, occurring mid-day. She has seen multiple providers for her headaches, but has been reluctant to try any medications due to concerns about side effects. She believes the headache symptoms were caused by changes in her sleep, and anxiety. Her headaches are described as follows: "headaches are immediate and are located in my temples but more severely in my right side. There is sensitivity to light and noise, and nausea. Nothing seems to make the headache go away until I go to sleep for the evening or take a nap." Her goal is to understand what is causing the headache and discuss headache management. Her biggest concern is that her headaches are more intense and not improving. Her past medical history includes anxiety and depression. She currently works as receptionist about 20 to 40 hours per week, and even though she rarely misses work, the headaches are starting to having major impact in her life as she is unable to function most days. She is very concerned about her well-being and spends significant amounts of her free time on the computer trying to research her symptoms. She has never had neuroimaging. The only medication she takes is acetaminophen.

What do I do now?

Diagnosis

Headache diagnoses are made mostly based on clinical characteristics and using the ICHD-3 diagnostic criteria. Duration of migraine episode without treatment is 4 or more hours. Patients with migraine have commonly associated symptoms such as light and sound sensitivity, and/or nausea.

This patient meets ICHD-3 diagnostic criteria of chronic migraine (CM). Chronic migraine is defined as headache occurring on 15 or more days/month for more than 3 months, which, on at least 8 days/month are migraine. The most common mistake that leads to missed diagnosis of CM is separating migraine and tension-type headaches and counting the days of each headache type separately (i.e., patient has 8 days of migraine and 8 days of tension-type headache per month) rather than counting them together as 16 headache days per month. The easiest approach to diagnosis is to lump migraine headache days and tension-type headache days and total them per month. Ask the patient to keep a headache diary and keep a record of total headache days per month and headache-free days per month, along with treatment days per month. Patients also tend to underreport, so it is good practice to also ask them how many days they have per month without any headache.

The differential diagnosis of CM also includes medication overuse headache (MOH), chronic tension–type headache, and New Daily Persistent Headaches, and these can often co-occur in the same patient. Patients with CM are at risk for MOH, which needs to be addressed to ensure the treatments prescribed are as effective as possible. Please see Chapter 27, "Day-in, Day-out" for more details.

Work-up

The next important step when evaluating patient with CM is to exclude a secondary cause of headache, particularly a treatable one such as neoplastic disease, vasculitis, idiopathic intracranial hypertension, and others. If the patient has a normal neurological examination and no other red flags, no further work-up is required for a patient with chronic migraine. Red flags include new-onset headache, worsening headaches, abnormalities on the neurological examination, fever, unintentional weight loss, and histories of cancer, transplant, or immunodeficiency. Patients with red flags or atypical presentations need further work-up with neuroimaging, such as magnetic resonance imaging (MRI) of the brain and lumbar puncture.

Treatment

Combining pharmacological acute and preventive treatment with lifestyle modifications, patient education, neuromodulation devices, and/or behavioral therapies is synergistic. We individualize the approach for each unique patient. Comorbidities should also be addressed to make the treatment more successful. For more details on lifestyle modifications, behavioral therapies, and complementary and integrative medicine therapies, please see Chapter 3, "The Answer is Not Always a Medicine."

ACUTE PHARMACOLOGICAL TREATMENT

Acute treatment should be started at the same time as preventive treatment, and patients need to be educated on the risk of developing MOH, as patients with CM often require acute treatments more than 10 days per month. We encourage providers to avoid prescribing opioids and butalbital, since they have high risk of MOH. The gold standard acute migraine treatment option are triptans. There are seven different triptans: almotriptan, eletriptan, frovatriptan, naratriptan, rizatriptan, sumatriptan, and zolmitriptan. Therapy with triptans can made more effective with added naproxen and/or dopamine antagonists. Triptans are contraindicated in patients with a history of cardiovascular disease and stroke.

If triptans are contraindicated or do not provide adequate relief, gepants or ditans can be used. Gepants are small-molecule calcitonin gene-related peptide (CGRP) receptor antagonists developed for the acute and preventive treatment of migraine. Gepants are not thought to cause MOH. Gepants are metabolized via CYP3A4, so potential drug–drug interactions have to be taken into account, and medication doses may need to be adjusted. Ubrogepant is available as a 50 mg to 100 mg pill to be taken at the start of the pain, and may be repeated once based on response and tolerability after ≥2 hours with a maximum of 200 mg per 24 hours. Rimegepant is available as a 75 mg orally disintegrating tablet as a single dose, maximum 75 mg/24 hours. It can be taken at the start of the pain or can be taken 15 days per month as a preventive option. Ditans have high affinity and selectivity for serotonin 5-HT1F receptors and lack the vasoconstrictor activity attributed to serotonin 5-HT1B receptor activated by triptans, so ditans can be used in patients with cardiovascular contraindications to triptans. Lasmiditan side effects include sedation and dizziness; patients must wait at least 8 hours between dosing and driving. Lasmiditan is available in 50 mg, 100 mg, or 200 mg PO as a single dose; maximum is 1 dose in 24 hours.

Other acute pharmacological treatments exist, such as dihydroergotamine mesylate (DHE), which is available as a nasal spray or intravenous injection.

PREVENTIVE PHARMACOLOGICAL TREATMENT

Preventive medication options include beta-blockers, anti-seizure medications, tricyclic antidepressants, and other therapies. Examples include topiramate, divalproex sodium, propranolol, candesartan, metoprolol, venlafaxine, duloxetine, amitriptyline, and memantine. OnabotulinumtoxinA (155–195 U) injections every 12 weeks are another FDA-approved treatment for the prevention of CM. It is a great option for patients who have difficulty taking daily oral preventive treatments or have intolerable side effects associated with oral medications. Newer preventive pharmacologic treatments include CGRP monoclonal antibodies (eptinezumab, fremanezumab, erenumab, and galcanezumab) and gepants (rimegepant and atogepant), which have shown efficacy in either phase 2 or phase 3 clinical trials in patients with CM. CGRP pathway inhibition is a disease-targeted approach to the prevention of migraine.

Galcanezumab is a humanized monoclonal antibody that selectively binds to and blocks the physiologic activity of CGRP. Erenumab and galcanezumab are both injected subcutaneously every month. Fremanezumab can be subcutaneously administered either monthly or every 3 months. Eptinezumab is given intravenously every 3 months. Atogepant is approved for the preventive treatment of migraine. It is to be taken every day and comes in 3 different doses (10 mg, 30 mg, and 60 mg tablets), which helps accommodate for potential drug–drug interactions seen between gepants and other medications metabolized through the CYP3A4 pathway. Rimegepant is also approved as 75 mg to be taken every other day as preventive treatment.

NEUROMODULATION

Neuromodulation devices are safe and effective acute and/or preventive treatment for chronic migraine. They should be considered in all patients, but especially in patients who prefer no pharmacotherapy or have had insufficient response or significant side effects or contraindications to medications. Two devices are FDA-approved for both acute treatment and preventive treatment: the transcutaneous supraorbital nerve stimulator (available over the counter) and the single pulse transcutaneous magnetic stimulator. Three devices are FDA-approved for the acute treatment of migraine: the remote electrical neuromodulation (REN) device, the noninvasive vagal nerve stimulator (VNS) device, and the combined occipital and trigeminal nerve stimulator.

KEY POINTS TO REMEMBER

- Think CM when patient has more than 15 days per month of any headaches for at least 3 months.
- To avoid missing diagnosis of CM, lump together migraine headache days and tension-type headache days, and total them per month.
- Ask patient to keep a headache diary and record total headache days per month and headache-free days per month, along with treatment days per month.
- There are many new treatment options available for both the acute and preventive treatment of CM.

Further Reading
1. Tepper D. "Gepants." *Headache.* 2020;60(5):1037–1039. https://doi.org/10.1111/head.13791
2. Ailani J, Burch RC, Robbins MS. "The American Headache Society consensus statement: Update on integrating new migraine treatments into clinical practice." *Headache.* 2021;61(7):1021–1039. https://doi.org/10.1111/head.14153
3. Becker WJ, Findlay T, Moga C, et al. "Guideline for primary care management of headache in adults." *Can Fam Physician.* 2015;61(8):670–679.
4. Pringsheim T, et al. "Canadian Headache Society guideline for migraine prophylaxis." *Can J Neurol Sci.* 2012;39(Suppl 2):S1–S59.

5. Buse DC, et al. "Migraine progression: A systematic review." *Headache.* 2019;59(3):306–338.

6. Buse DC, et al. "Sociodemographic and comorbidity profiles of chronic migraine and episodic migraine sufferers." *J Neurol Neurosurg Psychiatry.* 2010;81(4):428–432.

7. Lipton RB, et al. "Identifying natural subgroups of migraine based on comorbidity and concomitant condition profiles: Results of the chronic migraine epidemiology and outcomes (CaMEO) study." *Headache.* 2018;58(7):933–947. https://doi.org/10.1111/head.13342

8. Blech B, Starling AJ. "Noninvasive neuromodulation in migraine." *Curr Pain Headache Rep.* 2020;24(12):1–7.

9. Szperka CL, Ailani J, Barmherzig R, et al. "Migraine care in the era of COVID-19: Clinical pearls and plea to insurers." *Headache.* 2020;60(5):833–842.

10. Puledda F, Goadsby PJ. An update on nonpharmacological neuromodulation for the acute and preventive treatment of migraine. *Headache.* 2017;57(4):685–691.

11. Yuan H, Chuang TY. Update of neuromodulation in chronic migraine. *Curr Pain Headache Rep.* 2021;25(11):1–11.

7 From Shadows Down to the Abyss

Olivia Begasse de Dhaem and Carolyn Bernstein

Lucia is a 46-year-old right-handed woman who presents in late August to establish care after recently moving to the United States. She is very anxious, as she develops excruciating headaches that deform half of her face every September. The pain is so severe that she has considered putting an end to her life several times, but she is hanging on to her life because she is the only caretaker of her elderly mother who has Parkinson's disease. Although she enjoys a glass of red wine from time to time during the year, she cannot drink any alcohol in September, as it triggers her attacks. In her home country, she was admitted to the hospital many Septembers and given IV medications, but she does not remember the names. After about a month, the headaches subside, and she goes back to her regular life. She read about her symptoms and thinks she may have cluster attacks, but she was told these are most likely migraine because she is a woman.

What do I do now?

Diagnosis

The periodicity, unilaterality, facial autonomic symptoms, and severity of her attacks are concerning for cluster attacks. Although men are affected 3 times more than women, women can have cluster attacks. The first step is to gather more history. As shown in Table 7.1, Lucia's attacks meet the International Classification of Headache Disorders 3rd edition (ICHD-3) diagnostic criteria for cluster attacks.

Lucia has about 11 months of remission between the cluster periods, so she has episodic cluster headache. The majority (80%–85%) of patients with cluster attacks are episodic. Women tend to be more prone to being episodic, but the cluster periods tend to get longer with age. Of note, there have been years when Lucia did not develop any cluster attacks.

In addition to the characteristics of the attacks themselves, people with cluster attacks tend to have "shadows," a feeling before the attack that

TABLE 7.1 **ICHD-3 clinical characteristics of cluster headache compared to the characteristics of Lucia's attacks**

ICHD-3 diagnostic criteria	Lucia's attacks
At least 5 attacks	V
Severe or very severe unilateral orbital, supraorbital, and/or temporal pain lasting 15–180 minutes (when untreated)	Very severe, supraorbital, left-sided only, lasting about 30 minutes to 1 hour
Either or both of the following: 1. at least one of the following symptoms or signs, ipsilateral to the headache: —conjunctival injection and/or lacrimation —nasal congestion and/or rhinorrhea —eyelid edema —forehead and facial sweating —miosis and/or ptosis 2. a sense of restlessness or agitation	Left conjunctival injection, lacrimation, and eyelid edema. She cannot stand still during the attacks. The attacks often occur soon after she goes to bed, so she stands up and starts pacing around her bedroom.
Frequency between one every other day and 8 per day	She can have up to 3 attacks per day.

something is starting to happen, which is not necessarily painful; it can be a little facial twitch.

The differential diagnosis of cluster attacks includes other trigeminal autonomic cephalalgias, trigeminal neuralgia, cerebral aneurysm, brain tumor, and hypnic headaches.

She has had the same bouts of attacks for more than 20 years. She does not have any red flags. Her neurological examination is unremarkable. Secondary etiology is hence unlikely. Although it is typically taught that even common presentation of cluster attacks with no red flags warrant MRI and MRA of the brain, this often leads to incidental findings that don't impact management. Hence, it is reasonable to only image when red flags are present such as onset after 45 years old, attacks of prolonged duration, or any abnormalities on detailed neurological examination.

Management

Planning Ahead

Lucia was very smart and able to seek care in anticipation of her attacks. It is unfortunately not always possible for patients. When meeting patients with cluster attacks or possible cluster attacks, it is good to establish a treatment plan and obtain prior authorizations before the next attack. It is also good practice to make a follow-up appointment closer to the expected date of their cluster period to check in and plan for occipital nerve blocks. It is also important to discuss travels with patients, as altitude changes can bring on attacks.

Acute Treatment

The first step is to prescribe high-flow 100% oxygen at a rate of 12–15 liters per minute for 15 minutes through a firm plastic non-rebreathing facial mask. Patients hyperventilate quick short breaths, which may make them dizzy. Large M tanks can be used at home, and E tanks only when out of home. Another effective acute treatment for cluster is subcutaneous sumatriptan, which can be prescribed in 6 mg/0.5 mL syringes so the patients can choose whether they inject 3mg or 6mg at a time.

Bridge

Bridge therapy can be offered while waiting for preventive treatment to be effective. Bridge therapy includes ipsilateral greater occipital nerve block and a prednisone taper starting at 100 mg for 5 days and decreasing by 20 mg every 3 days.

Prevention

Galcanezumab 300 mg in 3 injections of 100 mg is approved for the treatment of episodic cluster attacks; it did not meet primary endpoints in the study for chronic cluster. Other preventive treatment includes verapamil, lithium, melatonin 10 mg nightly, or topiramate. It is also advisable that patients stop smoking tobacco. Verapamil has to be increased progressively while monitoring the EKG. The average dose tends to be 480 mg. There is also a vitamin D3 regimen developed by Pete Batcheller. The first step is to test the patient's 25(OH)D serum level. For refractory cluster attacks, other options include using occipital nerve stimulation and looking at whether the patient can enroll in a clinical trial, as other treatments are being evaluated such as ketamine and non-hallucinogen 2-bromo-lysergic acid diethylamide.

Support Network

Given the severity of the attacks, it is important discuss with empathy, ensure that patients have as many tools as possible, ask about their support system, inform them of support groups and the national suicide prevention line, and inform them about ways to reach you or someone on call at any time. Your notes have to be clear on the plans for an on-call provider to follow when the patient is in a cluster period. Cluster attacks can be very emotional and traumatic; some people may benefit from mental health treatment to deal with depression and/or post-traumatic stress disorder.

Further Evaluation

For patients with chronic cluster attacks, it may be worth doing a sleep study, as sleep-disordered breathing is associated with cluster attacks, and some patients have found relief with nasal continuous positive airway pressure.

- The first step is to perform a thorough history and neurological examination to make the diagnosis.
- People of all genders, races, and ethnicities can have cluster attacks. Children (even young children) can have cluster attacks. If the onset is >45 years old, please evaluate for secondary etiologies.
- It is important to be available for patients and ensure/work toward building a support network.
- A strong treatment plan should be in place with acute (at least high-flow oxygen and subcutaneous sumatriptan), bridge (prednisone and/or scheduling a greater occipital nerve block), and preventive treatment (such as galcanezumab, verapamil, melatonin, etc.).
- If the attacks are refractory to the treatment plan you feel comfortable offering, don't hesitate to reach out and refer to a headache specialist.

Further Reading

1. Pérez-Pereda S, Madera J, González-Quintanilla V, et al. "Is conventional brain MRI useful for the diagnosis of cluster headache in patients who meet ICHD-3 criteria? Experience in three hospitals in Spain." *J Neurol Sci.* 2021;434:120122. https://doi.org/10.1016/j.jns.2021.120122
2. Hattle AS. Cluster Attacks. A Guide to Surviving One of the Most Painful Conditions Known to Man. 2017. http://dx.doi.org/10.1038/d41586-020-02866-5
3. Obermann M, et al. "Safety and efficacy of prednisone versus placebo in short-term prevention of episodic cluster headache: a multicentre, double-blind, randomised controlled trial." *Lancet Neurol.* 2021;20(1):29–37.
4. Ornello R, et al. "Efficacy and safety of greater occipital nerve block for the treatment of cluster headache: a systematic review and meta-analysis." *Exp Rev Neurother.* 2020;20(11):1157–1167.
5. Goadsby PJ, et al. "Trial of galcanezumab in prevention of episodic cluster headache." *N Engl J Med.* 2019;381(2):132–141.
6. Dodick DW, et al. "Phase 3 randomized, placebo-controlled study of galcanezumab in patients with chronic cluster headache: Results from 3-month double-blind treatment." *Cephalalgia.* 2020;40(9):935–948.

7. Wilbrink LA, et al. "Safety and efficacy of occipital nerve stimulation for attack prevention in medically intractable chronic cluster headache (ICON): a randomised, double-blind, multicentre, phase 3, electrical dose-controlled trial." *Lancet Neurol.* 2021;20(7):515–525.

8. Newman LC. "Trigeminal autonomic cephalalgias." *Continuum.* 2015;21(4):1041–1057.

Looks Like a Stroke, Sounds Like a Stroke, But It's a . . .

Olivia Begasse de Dhaem and Carolyn Bernstein

Jane is a 19-year-old college student who has just returned from a semester abroad in Uganda. She has had menstrual migraine for years and has had several episodes of seeing a dark glowing spot in the middle of her visual field prior to developing a unilateral throbbing headache with sound and light sensitivity and nausea. She has come to see you for evaluation of her headaches after returning from her study abroad program.

On the day after she arrived in Uganda, she went running in the afternoon with a classmate on a dirt road in the small village where she was staying. The midday sun was bright, and she did not carry water with her on the run. She noticed after about 15 minutes that her left body was "dragging" and she felt weaker on the left. She slowed down but kept running; her vision then became cloudy and she was unable to see her classmate running on her left side. When she tried to tell him what was wrong, she could not get the correct words out, and sat down on the side of the road. She developed a severe throbbing headache. Her classmate was able to get help, and she was taken by ambulance to the nearest city where she had a CT scan of her brain that was reportedly normal, and was given intravenous medications but did not know what they were. The event resolved over about 6 hours, she felt fine, and did not have another similar episode during the four months of her study abroad program, although she did have several more headaches.

In the office, her medication list included ibuprofen for headaches and an estrogen/progesterone monophasic oral contraceptive pill (OCP) with 35 mcg of estrogen. Neurologic exam was entirely normal. She was not concerned about this event; her mother was quite worried and sought reassurance that it was not a stroke.

What do I do now?

Diagnosis

Jane's prior headaches meet the ICHD-3 criteria for migraine with aura: at least 2 episodes of fully reversible visual positive symptoms that gradually spread over 5 minutes and were followed by a headache within 60 minutes. The International Classification of Headache Disorders 3rd edition (ICHD-3) definition of migraine aura is based on the clinical characteristics of the aura and not of the headache.

The episode described lasted 6 hours, so it could be atypical aura. However, it is always very important to differentiate migraine aura from mimics such as transient ischemic attacks, seizure, carotid artery dissection, and arteriovenous malformations, and rule out secondary etiologies. Jane had arrived in Uganda that day, which makes malaria an unlikely etiology for that episode. Other considerations include reversible cerebral vasoconstriction syndrome (RCVS), especially given the heat and dehydration, multiple sclerosis, and syndrome of transient headache and neurological deficits with cerebrospinal fluid lymphocytosis (HaNDL). Cerebral amyloid angiopathy (CAA) should be on the differential diagnosis of new-onset "migraine" aura in elderly patients, as it can be a presentation of CAA transient focal neurological episode. Jane's brain MRI was normal.

Treatment

Current guidelines recommend the same acute and preventive treatment for migraine without and with aura.

There is currently no evidence-based treatment targeting the migraine aura specifically. Jane was prescribed rizatriptan ODT with naproxen as needed for her attacks of migraine with aura. Another good option for attacks of migraine with aura include aspirin as needed. Patients with migraine with aura may be slightly less responsive to sumatriptan (and maybe the other triptans) than patients with migraine without aura, but triptans still are commonly used. Triptans are usually to be taken at the onset of head pain and not at the onset of aura. However, some patients find that triptans (including subcutaneous sumatriptan) help with aura, so there is no reason for them not to try and take a triptan at the onset of their aura if it works for them.

There are no specific recommendations for preventive therapy for migraine with aura. There is some evidence that lamotrigine may be effective for reducing the aura frequency for migraine with aura, but there is no evidence for the use of lamotrigine for the prevention of migraine without aura.

MIGRAINE WITH AURA, ESTROGEN CONTRACEPTIVE AND HORMONAL REPLACEMENT, AND CARDIOVASCULAR RISK

Epidemiologic studies have demonstrated a mildly increased risk of stroke in patients with migraine with aura to about 18–40 in 100,000 person years; and estrogen-containing medications mildly increase this risk. The degree of increased risk is estrogen dose–dependent and not clearly known. In addition, other risk factors come into play such as age, smoking status, diabetes mellitus, hypertension, and other cardiovascular disease risk. There needs to be a risk-benefit discussion about contraception or other use of estrogen-containing agents with the patient and the provider who prescribed estrogen-containing agents in the first place. Given Jane's history of migraine with aura, the episode concerning for a secondary etiology, and other options for contraception, her estrogen-containing OCP was stopped. Jane's menstrual migraine now must be managed in another way than with continuous estrogen. Progesterone-only OCP tend to suppress aura and help with non-hormonal headaches, although more data is needed on drospirenone to see if it helps with menstrual migraine. For perimenopausal and menopausal women, a risk-benefit discussion addressing any potential contraindications and other risk factors is recommended before starting low-dose estrogen hormone replacement therapy. It is important to note that migraine with aura is NOT a contraindication to triptans, and triptans do not increase the cardiovascular risk of patients with migraine with aura.

MIGRAINE WITH AURA AND PATENT FORAMEN OVALE (PFO)

Migraine, and especially migraine with aura, is associated with a higher prevalence of PFO compared to the general population. PFO closure is not recommended for the management of migraine with aura.

- A careful history and physical examination are necessary, and sometimes further work-up as indicated, to rule out secondary etiologies and migraine aura mimics.
- Migraine aura mimics include transient ischemic attacks, seizure, carotid artery dissection, arteriovenous malformations, cerebral amyloid angiopathy, and transient focal neurological episodes.
- The management of migraine aura is similar to that of migraine without aura.
- Estrogen-containing agents slightly increase the cardiovascular risk (stroke, myocardial infarction) associated with migraine aura in a dose-dependent manner.
- Although migraine with aura is associated with PFO, it is not an indication for PFO closure by itself.

Further Reading

1. Weill A, Dalichampt M, Raguideau F, Ricordeau P, Blotiâŕe P, Rudant J, et al. "Low dose oestrogen combined oral contraception and risk of pulmonary embolism, stroke, and myocardial infarction in five million French women: cohort study." *BMJ.* 2016;353:i2002. https://doi.org/10.1136/bmj.i2002
2. Bousser MG, Conard J, Kittner S, et al. "Recommendations on the risk of ischaemic stroke associated with use of combined oral contraceptives and hormone replacement therapy in women with migraine. The International Headache Society Task Force on Combined Oral Contraceptive & Hormone Replacement Therapy." *Cephalalgia.* 2000;20:155–156.
3. Hansen JM, Charles A. "Differences in treatment response between migraine with aura and migraine without aura: lessons from clinical practice and RCTs." *J Headache Pain.* 2019;20(96). https://doi.org/10.1186/s10194-019-1046-4
4. Lebedeva ER, et al. "Explicit diagnostic criteria for transient ischemic attacks to differentiate it from migraine with aura." *Cephalalgia.* 2018;38(8):1463–1470. https://doi.org/10.1177/0333102417736901
5. Hansen JM, Goadsby PJ, Charles A. "Reduced efficacy of sumatriptan in migraine with aura vs without aura." *Neurology.* 2015;84(18):1880–1885.

9 Half of My Head Hurts

Saad Kanaan

Archibald is a 55-year-old man who presents with a 1-year history of headaches. Prior to that, he rarely had headaches and never had any severe headaches growing up.

The headache is constant in the right periorbital area and is described as mild to moderate aching pain at baseline but with episodes of severe, stabbing pain in the same location. During the severe episodes, he has right-sided photophobia, conjunctival injection, lacrimation, rhinorrhea, and profuse perspiration on the right forehead. He finds himself agitated and "pacing around" during the severe episodes. He has occasional "jolts" of pain in the same area lasting a few seconds. No nausea, vomiting, vision changes, or other focal neurologic symptoms. He has tried over-the-counter painkillers like acetaminophen and ibuprofen without relief. He does not have a family history of headache disorders. His neurologic examination during the baseline pain is unremarkable.

What do I do now?

Work-up

The most striking features from history are the presence of a chronic daily headache, the side-locked location of the headache in the distribution of the V1 (ophthalmic) division of the trigeminal nerve (Figure 9.1), and the presence of autonomic features ipsilateral to the headache. Archibald has several red flags: new headache after age 50, constant, and side-locked with autonomic features, so further work-up is warranted to rule out secondary causes of headache. A brain MRI with contrast is ordered to look

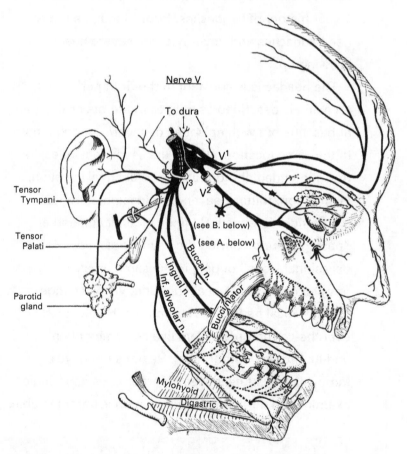

FIGURE 9.1 Anatomy of the trigeminal nerve including the V1 (ophthalmic), V2 (maxillary), and V3 (mandibular) divisions.

ADAPTED BY OXFORD UNIVERSITY PRESS

for a structural etiology such as a tumor, especially in the pituitary or posterior fossa. Traumatic brain injury is the most common cause of secondary hemicrania continua. An MRA of the head and neck is ordered to look for vascular lesions such as carotid dissection or cerebral aneurysm. Erythrocyte sedimentation rate and C-reactive protein are ordered to exclude temporal arteritis. In addition to a suggestion for temporal arteritis, elevated ESR in the case of advanced age, tobacco use, and constitutional symptoms warrant CT thorax to evaluate for potential lung carcinoma with vagal afferent stimulation. In Archibald's case, all those tests are unremarkable, hence a primary headache diagnosis is considered.

Diagnosis

The unilateral pain in the V1 ophthalmic division of the trigeminal nerve with ipsilateral autonomic symptoms and agitation/restlessness lead to the diagnosis of a trigeminal autonomic cephalalgia (TAC). Migraine is on the differential, as it can be unilateral and associated with autonomic symptoms.

The next step is to go through the definitions of the TACs and determine which one fits best with Archibald's case. Only one TAC presents with a constant daily headache: hemicrania continua. Hemicrania continua is characterized by a constant baseline, usually mild or moderate pain, with interspersed episodes of severe pain. The autonomic symptoms are more common during the severe episodes than the baseline pain. Chronic cluster headache may resemble hemicrania continua in that it is daily and is associated with episodes of severe headaches, but typically does not present with constant pain in between episodes. Chronic cluster headache does not respond to indomethacin.

According to the International Classification of Headache Disorders 3rd edition, hemicrania continua is diagnosed with the following criteria: (1) unilateral headache; (2) present for more than 3 months; (3) with either at least one autonomic sign ipsilateral to the headache (conjunctival injection and/or lacrimation, nasal congestion and/or rhinorrhea, eyelid edema, forehead and facial sweating, miosis and/or ptosis); a sense of restlessness/agitation/aggravation of the pain by movement; or both; and (4) absolute response to therapeutic doses of indomethacin.

The differential diagnosis currently includes the following:

1. Hemicrania continua, most likely, requires an absolute response to indomethacin
2. Chronic cluster headache with interictal pain
3. Chronic migraine
4. New daily persistent headache

The diagnosis of hemicrania continua is made mostly by history of a headache that meets the above criteria, exclusion of secondary causes, and an absolute response to indomethacin. Archibald needs to fully respond to the indomethacin trial to fulfill the diagnosis.

Treatment

Archibald is started on a trial of indomethacin as follows:

Days	Indomethacin Doses
1–3	25mg TID
4–6	50mg TID
7–21 or longer if needed	75mg TID

He is prescribed a proton pump inhibitor and warned about GI side effects of indomethacin.

Archibald calls excitedly that his headaches completely resolved when he titrated up to 50 mg 3 times daily, and therefore he did not have to increase it further. Patients are advised to continue the lowest effective dose. About 43% of patients show complete response to therapeutic dose of indomethacin after one week. Most patients need more than one week to show complete response, in which case therapeutic doses of indomethacin have to be continued for a longer duration. If the headache does not resolve on 225 mg daily of indomethacin, it is considered a failed trial. It is worth mentioning that parenteral indomethacin has also been used as a diagnostic test of hemicrania continua, but is not available in the United States. Once the pain is completely controlled, the dose of indomethacin should be reduced by 25 mg every 3 days until either the pain reappears or the patient gets completely off indomethacin. Some people may need to stay on a low dose of indomethacin. About 15% of patients have relapsing–remission course.

In order to decrease the use of indomethacin long term, other preventive medications can be considered such as topiramate 100–200mg (to be slowly titrated up), gabapentin (also to be titrated up), or amitriptyline 25mg (can be titrated up to 75mg). To date, there is only one case report on galcanezumab for hemicrania continua; more data is needed.

Epidemiology

The true prevalence of hemicrania continua is unknown given the fact that it is underdiagnosed, and patients can go years without an appropriate diagnosis. Delayed diagnosis and treatment can lead to months or years of suffering and disability.

KEY POINTS TO REMEMBER

- Diagnosis of hemicrania continua relies on careful history-taking, a high index of suspicion, and an absolute response to indomethacin.
- Secondary causes of hemicrania continua should be considered.
- Autonomic symptoms may be mild and not readily volunteered by patients.
- Indomethacin is the treatment of choice, and should be titrated up to headache freedom with a maximum daily dose of 225 mg daily.

Further Reading

1. Prakash S, et al. "Secondary hemicrania continua: Case reports and a literature review." *J Neurol Sci.* 2009;280(1-2):29–34. https://doi.org/10.1016/j.jns.2009.01.011
2. Prakash S, Patel P. "Hemicrania continua: clinical review, diagnosis and management." *J Pain Res.* 2017;10:1493–1509. https://doi.org/10.2147/JPR.S128472
3. González-Quintanilla V, et al. "First case of hemicrania continua responsive to galcanezumab." *Neurol Sci.* 2021;42(11):4775–4776. https://doi.org/10.1007/s10072-021-05476-9
4. Ashkenazi A, et al. "Hemicrania continua-like headache associated with internal carotid artery dissection may respond to indomethacin." *Headache.* 2007;47(1):127–130. https://doi.org/10.1111/j.1526-4610.2006.00637.x

5. Matharu MS, Cohen AS, McGonigle DJ, Ward N, Frackowiak RS, Goadsby PJ. "Posterior hypothalamic and brainstem activation in hemicrania continua." *Headache*. 2004;44(8):747–761. https://doi.org/10.1111/j.1526-4610.2004.04141.x
6. Antonaci F, Sjaastad O. "Hemicrania continua: towards a new classification?" *J Headache Pain*. 2014;15(1):8. https://doi.org/10.1186/1129-2377-15-8
7. Pareja JA, Caminero AB, Franco E, Casado JL, Pascual J, SÃnchez del RÃo M. "Dose, efficacy and tolerability of long-term indomethacin treatment of chronic paroxysmal hemicrania and hemicrania continua." *Cephalalgia*. 2001;21(9):906–910. https://doi.org/ 10.1046/j.1468-2982.2001.00287.x

10 Primary Stabbing Headache: "Sticking Out the Pain"

Shivang Joshi and Carly E. Harrington

A 49-year-old woman presents to the office expressing concern with regard to her new-onset headache symptoms, which started 3 months ago. She describes the pain as transient in nature, of such excruciating quality it feels as though she suddenly is being stuck with "a sharp stick" in her left eye. She notes that in her adolescence, she experienced tension-type headaches which were fairly tolerable and markedly different from her recent headaches. Her current symptoms, in comparison, are causing a significant degree of distress and disability in her daily activities, especially in her job performance.

As a waitress who must carry large and heavy trays of food, she sporadically experiences these headaches accompanied by a jolting pain that compels her to involuntarily close her eye and clutch the side of her head in agony. Her coworkers have been increasingly concerned with her condition, urging her to seek medical evaluation.

What do I do now?

Upon initial examination, the woman seems to be in otherwise good health, appropriately interacting, and manifesting no acute distress or pain. The patient describes each of her headaches in further detail as a single stabbing sensation resembling a "sharp stick being poked in [her] left eye a few times throughout the day." She notes that the single stab is severely painful with 8–9/10 intensity, localized to the left front-orbital area, and typically lasts only 5–8 seconds. The headaches are characterized as an intermittent pattern of sporadic stabs, irregular in both frequency and duration. Some days, she experiences only a single episode that lasts up to 8 seconds, while other days there may be only two or three episodes, each lasting only 5 seconds. These episodes have been occurring a few times per week over the past 3 months, with painful attacks never occurring more than 2 days consecutively.

The patient denies any head injuries, medication changes, exertional symptoms, autonomic features, and other clinical abnormalities. Upon review of her medical and social history, clinically relevant information includes previous tension-type headaches during adolescence and perimenopause, as well as a 20 pack-per-year history of tobacco use.

After careful history taking and a thorough neurological examination, many potential differential diagnoses arise. The diagnosis that may first be considered by clinicians given the patient's complaints is cluster headache. Diagnosed from detailed accounts of headache pain from the patient, cluster headaches exhibit classic characteristics of excruciating and severe unilateral orbital/supraorbital, and/or temporal pain lasting 15–180 minutes occurring with a frequency between every other day and 8 per day. These episodes of pain must also include the sense of restlessness with pain, or ipsilateral symptoms. For this patient, another diagnosis is more appropriate due to the short-lived nature of her headache symptoms and lack of ipsilateral symptoms.

Another headache disorder that closely mimics the characteristics described by the patient is that of primary thunderclap headache. Described as the "worst headache of one's life," primary thunderclap headache is a severe head pain with an abrupt onset reaching maximum intensity in less than 1 minute and lasting upwards of 5 minutes. This particular patient has never described her head pain as progressive, lasting longer than 8 seconds, or as the "worst headache of [her] life." Primary thunderclap headache seems unlikely.

Similar to the presentation of thunderclap headaches, reversible cerebral vasoconstriction syndrome (RCVS) also presents as a dramatic, sudden, and excruciating headache reaching maximum intensity in a matter of minutes. This patient has never experienced such pain, and presents with no neurological deficits nor any triggering factors for headache such as strenuous physical exertion, Valsalva maneuver, or acute stressful or emotional events.

Due to the patient's age, sex, and abrupt onset of symptoms, an MRI and MRA of the brain is warranted to rule out any secondary pathology that could be causing her complaints. Additional diagnostic testing should include ESR and CRP inflammatory laboratory testing to rule out giant cell arteritis (GCA). Temporal artery ultrasound is quite accurate in diagnosing GCA as well.

Another important referral is to ophthalmology for a dilated eye exam, given the patient reports of severe pain in the left orbital area as well as her long-standing history of smoking. Ophthalmic emergencies such as acute angle-closure glaucoma, which put the patient at risk for retinal vein occlusion, loss of vision, or permanent decreased visual acuity, should be identified early in the diagnostic testing.

Follow-up

The patient returns 4 weeks later for neurological reevaluation of her headache symptoms after obtaining all diagnostic testing ordered. MRI of the brain with and without contrast revealed microvascular ischemic changes with T2 hyperintensities, nonspecific findings related to aging and a history of tobacco use and headaches. MRA of the brain demonstrated unremarkable findings. The results of laboratory work revealed no signs of increased inflammatory markers, greatly decreasing clinical suspicion for GCA. Progress notes from the ophthalmologist were reviewed and reassuring that visual acuity and tonometry were within normal range.

As demonstrated in Table 10.1, the patient case, diagnostic testing, and information we have collected thus far is compared to the most appropriate diagnosis.

After analyzing the patient history, diagnostic imaging, and testing, primary stabbing headache is now the most appropriate diagnosis to establish. Primary stabbing headache, previously referred to as "ice-pick headache" and "needle-in-the-eye-syndrome," is a painful condition of infrequent and short-lived pain that mostly occurs in the extratrigeminal regions.

TABLE 10.1 **Working through the diagnosis**

Patient presentation	Diagnostic criteria
The patient has been experiencing a single stabbing sensation sporadically over the past 3 months, all of which lasted at least 5 seconds but never more than 8 seconds.	A. Head pain occurring spontaneously as a single stab or series of stabs and fulfilling criteria B and C. B. Each stab lasts up to a few seconds.
There is no pattern or identifiable frequency to track the stabbing attack. Some weeks she may experience the pain a few times a day while others a single episode.	C. Stabs recur with irregular frequency, from one to many per day.
The patient denies unilateral runny nose, stuffiness, monocular tearing, eye redness, droopy eyelid, or any other autonomic features.	D. No cranial autonomic symptoms.
Through diagnostic testing and careful history taking, giant cell arteritis, glaucoma, cluster headache, thunderclap headache, and reversible cerebral vasoconstriction syndrome have been ruled out.	E. No better accounted for by another ICHD-3 diagnosis.

Primary Stabbing Headache. The International Classification of Headache Disorders. https://ichd-3.org/other-primary-headache-disorders/4-7-primary-stabbing-headache/. Published February 6, 2018.

The dilemma that clinicians now face is whether or not to treat a condition with such infrequent, short-lived pain attacks with pharmacological or nonpharmacological measures. Treatment for primary stabbing headache is primarily based on patient tolerability and frequency of the attacks. Due to the short duration of pain, acute treatment may not be practical, and if attacks are infrequent then preventative medications may not be necessary.

If a patient is experiencing daily attacks, limiting ability to perform or function to their normal capacity, preventative medication may be appropriate. Common preventative medications that have been utilized for the prevention of primary stabbing headache include gabapentin, indomethacin, and other long-acting NSAIDs, as well as botox. Establishing preventative medications must be carefully deliberated both by the clinician and the patient. The patient must be cognizant that these painful attacks, which typically do not progress to any other more severe conditions nor influence morbidity, last only seconds compared to the potential for long-lasting adverse effects that may be experienced when on preventative medications. Ultimately, the clinical course must be dictated by the patient's tolerability of pain, lifestyle complications, job impairments, and adherence to medication regimen. Primary stabbing headaches have proven to be a debilitating headache condition requiring continued research to better optimize treatment options as well as enhance individual's well-being.

KEY POINTS TO REMEMBER

- Primary stabbing headache may closely mimic the characteristics of other headache disorders, making a detailed patient history of great importance to the clinician.
- Utilizing diagnostic testing such as MRI/MRA of the brain, laboratory testing including ESR and CRP, and results from a dilated eye exam by ophthalmologist allow the clinician to rule out any emergent conditions.
- Treatment for primary stabbing headache is largely dictated by the patient's tolerability of the pain and impact on their daily lives.

Further Reading

1. Ferrari MD, Haan J, Charles A, Dodick D, Sakai F. *Oxford Textbook of Headache Syndromes*. Oxford University Press; 2020.
2. Headache Classification Committee of the International Headache Society (IHS). The International Classification of Headache Disorders, 3rd edition. *Cephalalgia*. 2018;38:1–211.
3. Lee M, Chu MK, Lee J, Yoo J, Song HK. "Field testing primary stabbing headache criteria according to the 3rd beta edition of International Classification of Headache Disorders: a clinic-based study." *J Headache Pain*. 2016;17(1). https://doi.org/10.1186/s10194-016-0615-z
4. Primary Stabbing Headache. The International Classification of Headache Disorders. Published February 6, 2018: https://ichd-3.org/other-primary-headache-disorders/4-7-primary-stabbing-headache/
5. Singhal A, Rabinstein AA, Goddeau Jr DO, FAHA RP. Reversible cerebral vasoconstriction syndrome. In: Kasner, MD SE, ed. *UpToDate*.

11 Why Is the Alarm Clock Inside My Head?

Carolyn Bernstein and
Olivia Begasse de Dhaem

TM is a 60-year-old man, history of high cholesterol
but otherwise healthy and rarely seeks medical
attention. He presents with a 2-month description
of holocephalic headache that consistently wakes
him up from sleep at 3 a.m., "like the alarm is inside
my brain." The pain is global, moderately severe, no
tearing/rhinorrhea/ptosis/hidrosis/restlessness or any
other autonomic symptoms. He is not photophobic
or phonophobic, and has no numbness or weakness.
When he wakes with the pain, he will get up and go
into the bathroom (lights do not bother him when
he turns them on) and will take two Tylenol or some
aspirin, but this does not help much. He will sit up and
read or watch television, and the pain usually remits.
There is no family history of headache, and patient
did not have any trouble until several months ago. No
history of head trauma or recent illness or infection.
COVID 19 testing is negative. Neurologic exam is
completely normal.

What do I do now?

E xam is normal, headache has no red flags, and lab testing is normal. A new headache presentation in a patient over the age of 50 should prompt a thorough evaluation for secondary causes. Headaches attributed to intracranial neoplasia can be present in the morning and may have odd phenotypes. It is appropriate to image this patient; an MRI brain non-contrast is appropriate. Although description does not fit GCA (giant cell arteritis), it is prudent to check an ESR and a CRP level as well; you do not want to miss an entirely treatable cause of headache in this demographic. In addition, obstructive sleep apnea can cause nocturnal headache with early morning wakening; a sleep study is appropriate as well. Other secondary etiologies of nocturnal headaches include idiopathic intracranial hypertension, severe hypertension, hypercapnic respiratory failure, cervicogenic headache, withdrawal of analgesics, and delayed alcohol-induced headache. Once testing is completed, assuming all are normal, consider preventive medications. Since the headache presents "like clockwork," it is far better and likely more efficacious to use a nightly preventive therapy. Poor and interrupted sleep may have a myriad of health consequences regardless.

Once you have completed your work-up, assuming all is normal, this fits the description of hypnic headache. The old name was indeed "alarm clock headache." Patients are often relieved to have a diagnosis. These are the criteria: Recurrent headache attacks that develop only during sleep, and causing wakening. They must occur on at least 10 days per month for over three months, and last from 15 minutes to up to 4 hours after the patient wakes up. There can be no cranial autonomic features, and patient must not be restless. Note that this comports with your patient's description.

There is little evidenced treatment data. We suggest starting treatment with caffeine! Surprisingly, this may not interfere with sleep in an older population. Some patients report getting up to have a cup of coffee, but this defeats the point of treatment. Try caffeine tabs, low dose to begin with, prior to going to sleep. Melatonin is also a good choice; dose would be 5 mg. This may seem more intuitive; indeed, although the exact cause of hypnic headache is not known, it is felt to be related to some sort of circadian rhythm disturbance, and melatonin is often effective. Low-dose lithium can be used, as can indomethacin.

For many patients, having an accurate diagnosis can relieve anxiety around the headaches, and working to find an effective treatment is the next step. These are rare headaches but important to recognize and diagnose accurately.

PEARLS

1. Think of hypnic headache diagnosis when patients report consistent early morning wakening with headache.
2. Remember it is a "rule-out" diagnosis.
3. Explain the name and diagnostic criteria to your patients for validation.
4. Not many evidenced medications exist, but try caffeine or melatonin as first-line options.

Further Reading
1. Lanteri-Minet M. "Hypnic headache." *Headache.* 2014;54(9):1556–1559. https://doi.org/10.1111/head.12447
2. Holle D, Naegel S, Obermann M. "Hypnic headache." *Cephalalgia.* 2013;33(16):1349–1357. https://doi.org/10.1177/0333102413495967
3. Holle D, Obermann M. "Hypnic headache and caffeine." *Expert Rev Neurother.* 2012;12(9):1125–1132. https://doi.org/10.1586/ern.12.100

12 My Head Hurts Everyday

Jessica Gautreaux

Gaspar is a 17-year-old boy who comes to your clinic accompanied by his mother for evaluation for headaches. He has been suffering from one long headache that just has not gone away for the last 6 months. He remembers that it was there when he woke up on the morning of March 3. He describes the headache as "all over" and varying from squeezing to pounding. It is always present and usually moderate in intensity, but can fluctuate in severity. He has noted that when the pain is severe, he is light-sensitive and has to stop what he is doing. His mom recalls that he was experiencing cold symptoms at the time the headache started. At first she thought the head pain was related to the cold, but it then persisted after his other symptoms resolved. She herself has migraine, but her son never had a headache like hers. Gaspar has anxiety, which he feels has been worse lately because he is worried that something "serious" is going on.

What do I do now?

Diagnosis

Gaspar is describing head pain with features suggestive of new daily persistent headache (NDPH). He clearly recalls the onset of this daily, unremitting headache. The features of the headache such as quality, severity, and associated symptoms vary, but what is distinct is the fact that this headache began in a patient with no headache history and had been continuous since a very clear onset.

As with most headache disorders, a detailed and accurate history is the most important factor in making an accurate NDPH diagnosis. Most often, NDPH occurs in those with no prior headache history. The International Classification of Headache Disorders 3rd edition (ICHD-3) does not define any specific features of the head pain or associated symptoms in its criteria for diagnosis of NDPH. The pain is usually bilateral, moderate in intensity, and constant. NDPH often has features of either migraine or tension-type headache, and patients describe a myriad of associated symptoms such as sleep disturbances, vertigo, blurred vision, difficulty with concentration, fatigue. The ICHD-3 diagnostic criteria include a distinctly remembered onset of continuous unremitting pain for 24 hours, which has persisted for at least 3 months. A limitation is that the recall of the date of onset is variable from 20% to 100%. However, it is important to clarify the headache characteristics when taking a history to differentiate NDPH from other chronic daily headache conditions such as chronic migraine, chronic tension-type headache, medication overuse headache, or hemicrania continua.

Gaspar's headache fluctuates and at times is severe and pulsatile with photohobia and phonophobia, which fulfills criteria for chronic migraine. However, given the clearly remembered sudden onset and unremitting character, NDPH is the better diagnosis for him. It is imperative to differentiate NDPH from hemicrania continua in a patient presenting with a new, chronic daily headache, as hemicrania continua is very responsive to treatment with indomethacin. As discussed further in Chapter 9, "Half of My Head Hurts," hemicrania continua is characterized by a continuous, unilateral headache that fluctuates in intensity and is associated with either autonomic symptoms ipsilateral to the headache or a sense of restlessness or agitation.

In patients who have a preexisting headache disorder, it is important to define whether there was a sudden change in their headache pattern, or if they had a gradual increase in the frequency of their headache attacks. A gradual worsening of their headache frequency suggests either a transformation from the episodic to the chronic form of their preexisting headache disorder, or medication overuse headache (MOH) and makes NDPH unlikely. To distinguish MOH from NDPH, it is important to ask whether the patient increased their acute medication use in response to developing a new daily headache (NDPH), or if they have progressively been using more acute treatments in attempt to address their preexisting headache disease (MOH). If episodic attacks of their primary headache disorder suddenly become persistent and unremitting one day, and all potential secondary etiologies for this acute change are excluded, then NDPH may be the best diagnosis.

Work-up

A new-onset, unremitting headache or an acute change from a preexisting headache disease are red flags and warrant further investigation. Any systemic or neurological symptoms or signs found during the clinical evaluation may further guide work-up. All patients with NDPH should be evaluated with brain MRI with gadolinium contrast (if no contraindications to MRI and/or contrast). In some patients, MRA/MRV may be warranted as well. For example, a patient with a hypercoagulable state may need a head MRV to rule out a cerebral venous thrombosis. Head and neck MRA may be warranted if there is any concern for carotid or vertebral dissections in the case of neck trauma, for example. NDPH can be a presentation of intracranial pressure abnormalities. If there is papilledema on exam, or there is a concern for central nervous system infection, a lumbar puncture with opening pressure and cerebrospinal fluid analysis should be performed. Both idiopathic intracranial hypertension and intracranial hypotension can also lead to an NDPH presentation; thus it may be necessary to rule out a spontaneous cerebrospinal fluid leak.

Epidemiology

The estimated prevalence of NDPH is 0.03%–0.1%. It is more common in women than men, and more common in children/adolescents than adults. It can present at any age, with cases reported in those >70 years old. Mood disorders such as depression and anxiety are more prevalent in patients with NDPH; these comorbidities should be screened for and addressed.

Pathophysiology

Little is known about the pathogenesis of NDPH. Many patients report a precipitating event for their NDPH with infection or flu-like illness being most commonly reported, even more so in children. Stressful life events, surgical procedures, and other triggers have been described. Associations with EBV have been suggested and studied, but it is speculative for now. Controlled studies are still needed to better understand the mechanism behind NDPH. The lack of understanding of the pathogenesis of the disease limits the development of specific treatments for the disorder.

Prognosis

NDPH is one of the most refractory primary headache disorders, and there is currently a lack of double-blind placebo-controlled trials to guide therapy. There is very limited improvement even with aggressive treatment. There are case reports of NDPH lasting >20 years despite aggressive treatments. Some reports suggest that early treatment of NDPH in the first 3–12 months from onset results in better treatment outcomes.

In a recent retrospective review of patients being treated for NDPH, three patterns were noted:

1. A persisting form, where the headache was unremitting from onset. Most patients experienced continuous daily head pain for >24 months.
2. A remitting form, where headache frequency improved to a rate of no more than 4 headache days per month. Remission occurred within 24 months.
3. A relapsing–remitting form, where patients experienced periods of headache remission then return of their NDPH. The first remission occurred within 24 months.

Treatment

Most headache specialists treat NDPH based on the headache phenotype, for example using migraine treatments if migraine features are present.

Small studies have looked at methylprednisolone, tetracycline derivatives, topiramate, gabapentin, mexilitine, nerve blocks, OnabotuliumtoxinA, intravenous lidocaine, intravenous dihydroergotamine, intravenous ketamine, nimodipine, combination therapies, and osteopathic manipulation in NDPH.

At the time of diagnosis, it is important to discuss the diagnosis, approach to treatment, and prognosis of NDPH with patients. Counseling patients on goals for treatment and expectations for treatment is paramount for NDPH. Due to the refractory nature of the headache itself, many headache medicine specialists focus on ways to improve quality of life for patients with NDPH. Helping patients to preserve functionality and to cope with a diagnosis of pain refractory to treatment is important in NDPH and may require a multidisciplinary approach including psychologists and physical therapists.

KEY POINTS TO REMEMBER

- NDPH is an entity that is important to recognize clinically.
- Patients can typically pinpoint the very day that NDPH began.
- NDPH may have the features of chronic migraine or chronic tension-type headache, but if criteria for NDPH are met, then the diagnosis is NDPH.
- It is important to differentiate NDPH from hemicrania continua, which is treatable with indomethacin.
- Secondary headaches should be ruled out with appropriate investigations.
- There is no specific treatment for NDPH. Treatment is tailored based on the features of the headache in each specific patient, though it is recognized that NDPH is often refractory to current headache treatment options. There is some suggestion that early treatment might produce a better response to treatment.

Further Reading

1. Begasse de Dhaem O, Rizzoli PR. "Refractory headaches (MOH, NDPH)." *Seminars on Headache,* 2022.

2. Rozen TD. "Triggering events and new daily persistent headache: age and gender differences and insights on pathogenesis-a clinic-based study." *Headache.* 2016;56(1):164–173.

3. Robbins MS, Evans RW. "The heterogeneity of new daily persistent headache." *Headache.* 2012;52(10):1579–1589. https://doi.org/10.1111/j.1526-4610.2012.02280.x

4. Riddle EJ, Smith JH. "New daily persistent headache: a diagnostic and therapeutic odyssey." *Curr Neurol Neurosci Rep.* 2019;19(5):21.

5. Robbins MS, Grosberg BM, Napchan U, Crystal SC, Lipton RB. "Clinical and prognostic subforms of new daily-persistent headache." *Neurology* 2010;74(17):1358–1364. Published correction appears in *Neurology.* 2010;75(18):1660.

6. Evans RW, Seifert TD. "The challenge of new daily persistent headache." *Headache.* 2011;51(1):145–154.

7. Yamani N, Olesen J. "New daily persistent headache: a systematic review on an enigmatic disorder." *J Headache Pain.* 2019;20:80. https://doi.org/10.1186/s10194-019-1022-z

13 Let's Talk About Jaw Overuse

María F. Hernández-Nuño de la Rosa

Jane is a 55-year-old woman who presents with a chief complaint of right temple headache. The pain began around 3 months ago with no particular event associated with its onset and has gradually worsened since then. It is continuous and dull in nature but becomes sharp with jaw function. The pain increases as the day progresses, ranging between 2/10 in the morning upon awakening and 7/10 toward the end of the day. She does not have any visual, motor, or sensory disturbances nor any photophobia, phonophobia, nausea, or vomiting. However, she has persistent muscle stiffness in the face and points to the ipsilateral masseter area. She has difficulty opening her mouth but does not experience any joint sounds or any episodes of jaw locking. On examination, her chief complaint is elicited upon palpation of the right temporalis muscle. The ipsilateral masseter muscle is tender, and limited mouth opening is present. Signs of severe attrition are found upon examination of the oral cavity.

What do I do now?

Temporomandibular disorders (TMDs) are a group of musculoskeletal disorders with a high prevalence in the general population, particularly in women. They affect the masticatory muscles, the temporomandibular joint, and the associated structures, provoking a variety of sign and symptoms such as pain, joint sounds, and limited mandibular range of motion, as well as difficulty in mastication and/or in speech. With a multifactorial pathogenesis, a detailed history and physical examination and an imaging study both help achieve the correct diagnosis and guide the most appropriate management approach. In addition, performing a comprehensive psychosocial assessment in patients with suspected TMD is paramount for the clinician to identify parafunctional habits and life stressors that might have precipitated and/or might have contributed to perpetuate this condition.

Diagnosis

The Diagnostic Criteria for Temporomandibular Disorders (DC/TMD), a validated screening and diagnostic tool, describes the 12 most common types of TMD: myalgia, local myalgia, myofascial pain, myofascial pain with referral, headache attributed to TMD, arthralgia, four disc-related disorders, degenerative joint disease, and subluxation. This classification defines headache attributed to TMD as a headache in the temple area secondary to a concomitant TMD that can be modified by jaw function or parafunction, and in which provocation testing of the masticatory system replicates the pain. It requires the patient to present a positive history for both of the following: (1) a headache of any type in the temple during the last 30 days that (2) can be modified with jaw function or parafunction. In addition, the exam should be positive for both of the following criteria: (1) confirmation of the headache location in the area of the temporalis muscle(s) as well as (2) report of familiar headache in the temple area upon provocation testing via (a) palpation of the temporalis muscle(s) and/or (b) maximum unassisted or assisted opening, right or left lateral, or protrusive movement(s). The International Classification of Headache Disorders 3rd edition (ICHD-3) lists headache attributed to TMD as a subtype of secondary headaches.

History Taking

More information should be obtained on history to formally diagnose Jane with headache attributed to TMD. Her pain is aggravated by jaw function and significantly worse at end of the day, which suggests the presence of a TMD. However, the clinician should ask more information on what type of activities typically intensify the symptoms. Jane is currently on a soft diet as she is unable to chew hard foods, and she has difficulty talking for long periods of time. At this point, and given Jane's age, it is important to discuss with her the difference between pain and jaw claudication (a combined feeling of discomfort and tiredness). Jane does not have any visual disturbances or jaw claudication. However, the threshold to screen for giant cell arteritis with ESR in patients with new-onset temporal headaches after age 50, like Jane, should be low. The palpation exam on the ipsilateral temporal artery is unremarkable, and her ESR and CRP values are within normal limits.

REFERRAL TO AN OROFACIAL PAIN SPECIALIST

Jane is referred to an orofacial pain specialist who performs a thorough temporomandibular joint and masticatory muscle assessment, including provocation testing, to confirm the presence of a TMD. In addition, the orofacial pain specialist investigates further whether parafunctional habits such as bruxism, as well as potential life stressors, might be playing a role in the etiology of her chief complaint. Given that Jane hardly feels any pain in the morning upon awakening, it is suspected that she may have a mandibular parafunctional habit, unconsciously or consciously, during the day. Jane clenches her teeth constantly during her work hours, but barely on the weekends, and has already cracked a molar. She also chews gum compulsively and has been under a high level of stress at work since she was promoted a few months ago.

Furthermore, a battery of standardized and validated questionnaires should be routinely used for behavioral screening (see Table 13.1). Jane screens positive for severe anxiety (GAD-7 = 16) and poor sleep quality (PSQI = 5).

TABLE 13.1 Commonly used questionnaires for behavioral screening

Domain	Questionnaire	Number of items
Anxiety	General Anxiety Disorder-7 (GAD-7)	7
Depression	Patient Health Questionnaire (PHQ-9)	9
PTSD	PTSD Checklist (PCL-5)	20
Sleep quality	Pittsburgh Sleep Quality Index (PSQI)	19, distributed in 7 components

Imaging

It is recommended to order a panoramic radiograph of the temporomandibular joint to rule out any underlying bony pathology that might be referring pain to the temporalis muscle. Jane's radiograph is unremarkable.

Treatment

A self-management program to prevent further injury to the masticatory system is established for Jane. It includes voluntary limitation of the mandibular function and gentle stretching exercises and massage of the masticatory muscles to be performed at home, along with heat therapy. If this strategy is not enough to alleviate her symptoms, a course of physical therapy and pharmacotherapy consisting of a combination of an anti-inflammatory and a muscle relaxant should be prescribed. This will include a trial of meloxicam 15 mg once a day in the morning for no longer than 2 weeks, along with cyclobenzaprine 10 mg to be taken at bedtime for a maximum of 3 weeks. Furthermore, an intraoral orthotic device to be used overnight and intermittently during the day is also recommended. Awareness and modification of mandibular parafunctional habits like teeth-clenching and chewing gum compulsively are initially addressed with patient education and feedback mechanisms such as an alarm in the phone, or sticky notes strategically placed at home and at work. However, given that Jane screened positive for severe anxiety and poor sleep quality, she is referred to a clinical psychologist for further evaluation and management with cognitive behavioral therapy. In case of refractory pain, the use of trigger point or even botulinum toxin injection therapy should be considered.

Prognosis

A satisfactory prognosis of Jane's headache is expected as long as her TMD symptoms are well controlled. Addressing her anxiety and mandibular parafunctional habits is important to achieve the best results.

KEY POINTS TO REMEMBER

- Temporomandibular disorders (TMDs) are a heterogeneous group of musculoskeletal disorders that affect the masticatory muscles, the temporomandibular joint, and the associated structures. They have a high prevalence in the general population, particularly in women, and present a multifactorial pathophysiology.
- The Diagnostic Criteria for Temporomandibular Disorders (DC/TMD) and the International Classification of Headache Disorders 3rd edition (ICHD-3) are two validated tools for the screening and diagnosis of headache attributed to TMD.
- Parafunctional habits of the mandible such as bruxism, in some cases secondary to persistent life stressors, might play a critical role in the etiology of this condition. Thus, the use of standardized and validated questionnaires for behavioral screening as part of a comprehensive psychosocial assessment is recommended.
- A multimodal treatment plan involving a combination of a self-management program, physical therapy, pharmacotherapy, and an intraoral orthotic device is recommended for TMDs. A referral to a clinical psychologist might also be needed. For refractory pain, trigger point or even botulinum toxin injection therapy are used.
- A thorough differential diagnosis should be performed to rule out the presence of giant cell arteritis, a condition that untreated can lead to blindness.

Further Reading

1. Scrivani SJ, Keith DA, Kaban LB. "Temporomandibular disorders." *N Engl J Med.* 2008;359(25):2693–2705.
2. Schiffman E, Ohrbach R, Truelove E, et al. "Diagnostic criteria for temporomandibular disorders (DC/TMD) for clinical and research applications: recommendations of the International RDC/TMD Consortium Network* and Orofacial Pain Special Interest Groupdagger." *J Oral Facial Pain. Headache.* 2014;28(1):6–27.
3. de Leeuw R, Klasser G, American Academy of Orofacial Pain. *Orofacial Pain: guidelines for assessment, diagnosis and management.* 6th ed. Hanover Park, IL: Quintessence Publishing; 2018.
4. Khawaja SN, Scrivani SJ, Holland N, Keith DA. "Effectiveness, safety, and predictors of response to botulinum toxin type A in refractory masticatory myalgia: a retrospective study." *J Oral Maxillofac Surg.* 2017;75(11):2307–2315.

14 My Right Eye Is On Fire

Olivia Begasse de Dhaem

Jane is a 30-year-old-woman with a history of episodic migraine with visual aura who now presents with new right eye pain.

Usually, her visual aura scotomas are followed by throbbing pain in the distribution of the right supratrochlear nerve, which progressively spreads to the right retroorbital and frontal regions. She has had long-standing constant photophobia waxing and waning in severity and worsened by night driving. She has worn contact lenses for myopia for 20 years with no recent changes. She never had eye pain before. She did not have any trauma to the eye.

One morning, she woke up with new-onset severe right eye pain. The pain has been constant since, but is worst in severity in the morning upon waking up. The eye pain is burning in character. Exposure to bright lights and her visual aura scotomas worsen the eye pain, too. The eye pain and her attacks of migraine with visual aura seem to trigger each other. An ophthalmology exam in the emergency room was unremarkable.

What do I do now?

J ane was asked to refrain from wearing contact lenses until the pain improved and to use preservative-free artificial tears 3 times daily. Although the lubricant eye gel she used made her vision blurry, its application was not painful, contrary to the artificial tears. She was also advised to increase omega-3 in her diet.

Upon evaluation by a neurologist, the history did not suggest a central process and the exam was unremarkable. There was no afferent pupillary defect, proptosis, Horner's syndrome, or papilledema. Her neurologist performed a right supratrochlear nerve block with 1:1 ratio of 0.5cc of 0.75% bupivacaine and 0.5cc of 2% lidocaine. Given her ocular neuropathic pain and increased frequency in migraine attacks, Jane was prescribed her 10 mg amitriptyline nightly both for mitigation of her disabling eye pain and for migraine prevention. Other considerations for neuropathic corneal pain include systemic gabapentin, pregabalin, carbamazepine, nortriptyline, low-dose naltrexone, or sterile compounded topical 0.1% lacosamide.

Upon evaluation by the ophthalmologist, Jane completed the ocular pain assessment survey (OPAS), a validated tool to quantify and monitor corneal pain. Her fundoscopic exam and eye pressure were unremarkable. Jane did not report decreased visual acuity in bright lights nor darkness, which would be concerning for a retinal etiology. Eye pressure is important because glaucoma can cause photophobia and pain. The meibomian glands should be evaluated, as their dysfunction can contribute to dry eye symptoms. The ocular surface slit-lamp examination with fluorescein showed corneal neovascularization but no evidence of prior trauma. A careful slit-lamp exam helps rule out conditions like epithelial basement membrane dystrophy, which causes morning eye pain. The Schirmer test was positive on the right eye (2mm), and upon further examination Jane had dry mouth on exam. Upon further questioning, she did not have any other symptoms of rheumatologic, endocrinologic, or dermatologic symptoms. She did have autonomic symptoms such as heat intolerance, minimal sweating, orthostatic lightheadedness, and nausea. Jane's peripheral pain and allodynia were confirmed with topical 0.5% proparacaine stopping her right eye pain, and 5% normal saline drops triggering severe burning pain in the right eye only, which then subsided with numbing drops, respectively. Feeling of eye dryness without objective evidence of dry eyes and with photophobia and no abnormalities on regular ophthalmologic exam suggest corneal neuropathy.

Confocal microscopy showed a corneal neuroma in the right eye. Risk factors for corneal neuroma and corneal neuropathic pain include migraine, prolonged contact lens wear, and autoimmune disease. Blood work was sent (TS-HDS IgM, FGFR3 IgG, tissue transglutaminase antibody, CBC, BMP, LFT, TSH, ACE, B2, B12, D25, ANCA, ESR, CRP, serum protein electrophoresis, immunoglobulin panel, ANA, rheumatoid factor, gliadin, ENA SSA and SSB) and came back positive for rheumatoid factor and SSA, and low B2. Riboflavin supplementation was recommended, and Jane was referred to rheumatology for further evaluation and management. To address the corneal neovascularization, the ophthalmologist advised her not wearing contact lenses until the pain improved. At which time, an appointment with an optometrist would be recommended to advise on the safest possible contact lens.

In addition to work-up and management of underlying issues, twice daily topical cyclosporine 0.05% drops and a short course of topical loteprednol gel were prescribed. Loteprednol 0.5% gel penetrates the eye less and has a lower concentration of the neurotoxic preservative benzalkonium chloride than other topical corticosteroids. Jane preferred the gel to the suspension, as the gel application was calming her eye pain even though it was blurring her vision a bit. People with very severe allodynia might not tolerate the preservative in loteprednol and may be more comfortable with sterile, preservative-free compounded topical methylprednisolone 1%. Loteprednol gel is prescribed as a slow taper of 4 times daily for 2 weeks, then twice daily for 2 weeks, and finally once daily over 6 to 12 weeks. Jane's steroid-sparing anti-inflammatory topical treatment was chosen based on her copay at the pharmacy with the coupons she had, but alternative options included lifitegrast 5% and tacrolimus 0.03%. The choice of topical agent may be a process of trial and error based on patients' response to their preservatives.

For Jane, the loteprednol and cyclosporine provided partial relief, so autologous serum tears were also started two months later, which significantly helped with pain relief. Autologous serum tears contain neurotrophic growth factors that help tear film stability in severe dry eye, the Schirmer's scores, photoallodynia, allodynia, corneal subbasal nerve density, and corneal epithelial healing. During that time, Jane also made behavioral changes such as avoiding driving at night, using natural light instead of fluorescent light, and frequently wearing sunglasses. The concept of dark adaptation and the potential worsening of light sensitivity with reduced exposure to light was discussed, as well as FL-41 tint glasses to reduce exposure to blue light.

A year later, Jane's eye pain was managed with daily autologous serum tears and riboflavin for prevention. The autologous serum tear application was progressively reduced from 8 times daily to daily. Jane's pain upon application due to the cold temperature of the serum tears progressively subsided. Given the improvement in her eye pain, next line treatments such as cryopreserved amniotic membrane or scleral lenses were not considered.

For acute breakthrough right eye burning pain, Jane was prescribed topical nepafenac 0.3% eye drops PRN. She tried other topical NSAID eye drops PRN, but their application worsened her pain. Treating her attacks of right eye pain early both aborts her eye pain and prevents its evolution into a migraine attack. Whether the eye pain triggered her migraine attacks, or the worsening photophobia during the prodromal phase of her migraine attack led to eye pain was unknown, but it was worth trying to treat the preceding eye pain with a topical agent. It worked; it prevented the worsening of eye pain into a full-blown migraine attack for Jane. The bidirectional relation between Jane's migraine attacks, supratrochlear pain, and right eye pain makes sense from an anatomical point of view, as the trigeminal nerve is involved in all three. The ophthalmic (V1) trigeminal nerve branches include its tentorial branch (which provides dural innervation), the frontal nerve (from which the supratrochlear nerve arises), and the nasociliary nerve. The ciliary nerves arise from the nasociliary nerve and innervate the cornea. Regarding photophobia, light sensitivity, and eye pain, Dr. Noseda and colleagues identified in rodents a direct pathway between the intrinsically photosensitive retinal ganglion cells (IPRGCs) and thalamic nuclei involved in somatosensation and pain (posterior, lateral posterior, and intergeniculate), which also process painful trigeminal information from the dura. It is important to validate patients' symptoms and describe some of the anatomy to them.

The prognosis of neuropathic eye pain is variable and partially depends on other comorbidities including other chronic pain and mood disorders, which should be addressed. Early treatment is important. Dry eye symptoms (such as burning, dryness, foreign body sensation, photoallodynia, irritation) negatively impact the visual quality of life of people with migraine. Without objective findings of eye dryness (basal tear secretion, corneal sensitivity, tear film break-up time, tear osmolarity, Schirmer test), those symptoms are hypothesized to be related to the reduced corneal nerve fiber density observed in patients with chronic migraine.

Neuropathic corneal pain can be due to local causes (such as ocular surgery, trauma, or infection), or systemic causes (such as small-fiber polyneuropathy or an autoimmune condition such as lupus). Treatment approaches

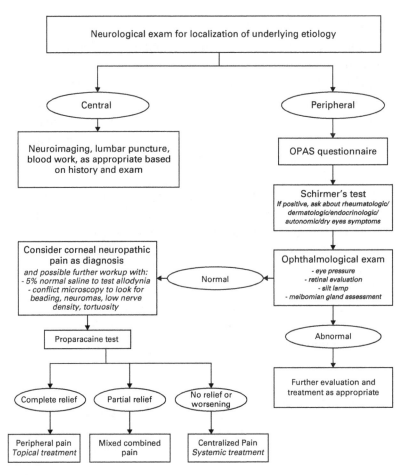

FIGURE 14.1 Clinical Approach to Eye Dryness Symptoms (e.g., burning, irritation, etc.) and Photophobia.

will differ based on whether the pain is peripheral, central, or mixed. Topical treatments will be preferred for peripheral pain initially. Systemic treatments can be helpful for peripheral sensitization. Systemic treatments with tricyclics, for example, will be preferred initial treatments for central pain. Sometimes, as it is the case with Jane, there is a mixed pain with ocular surface burning pain, supratrochlear pain, and headache all interrelated.

Dry eye symptoms are common and disabling. They warrant further evaluation for diagnosis and treatment. Figure 14.1 summarizes the approach.

KEY POINTS TO REMEMBER

- The first step with eye pain and photophobia is to localize the lesion through history and examination: central, peripheral, or systemic. Work-up and management will depend on localization. For example, if the exam reveals an afferent pupillary defect, optic neuritis must be considered. If the neurological exam is unremarkable and a peripheral cause is suspected, a thorough ophthalmological evaluation is needed to look for ocular etiologies.
- Dry eye symptoms are common and disabling in people with chronic migraine. The symptoms of dry eyes such as burning pain and irritation may not be correlated with objective findings. This may be due to morphological changes in corneal innervation.
- Corneal neuropathic pain is suggested by (1) subjective symptoms of dry eyes, (2) no objective evidence of dry eyes, (3) photophobia, (4) no abnormalities on regular ophthalmologic exam.

Further Reading
1. Digre KB, Brennan KC. "Shedding light on photophobia." *J Neuroophthalmol.* 2012;32(1):68–81. https://doi.org/10.1097/WNO.0b013e3182474548
2. Dieckmann G, et al. "Neuropathic corneal pain: approaches for management." *Ophthalmology.* 2017;124(11S):S34–S47. https://doi.org/10.1016/j.oph tha.2017.08.004

3. Celebi AR, Ulusoy C, Mirza GE. "The efficacy of autologous serum eye drops for severe dry eye syndrome: A randomized double-blink crossover study." *Graefes Arch Clin Exp Ophthalmol.* 2014;252(4):619–626.

4. Jirsova K, Brejchova K, Krabcova I, et al. "The application of autologous serum eye drops in severe dry eye patients; subjective and objective parameters before and after treatment." *Curr Eye Res.* 2014;39(1):21–30.

5. Aggarwal S, Colon C, Kheirkhah A, Hamrah P. "Efficacy of autologous serum tears for treatment of neuropathic corneal pain." *Ocul Surf.* 2019;17(3): 532–539. https://doi.org/10.1016/j.jtos.2019.01.009

6. Kinard K, et al. "Chronic migraine is associated with reduced corneal nerve fiber density and symptoms of dry eye." *Headache.* 2015;55(4): 543–549. https://doi.org/10.1111/head.12547

7. Ozudogru S, et al. "Reduced visual quality of life associated with migraine is most closely correlated with symptoms of dry eye." *Headache.* 2019;59(10): 1714–1721. https://doi.org/10.1111/head.13662

8. Noseda R, et al. "Migraine photophobia originating in cone-driven retinal pathways." *Brain.* 2016;139(Pt 7): 1971–1986. https://doi.org/10.1093/brain/aww119

Severe Facial Pain in the Emergency Department

Carrie E. Robertson

A 59-year-old man presents with a one-year history of worsening facial pain. He describes shooting, electrical shock–like pain in the right cheek, upper gums, and upper lip, especially right by his nose. Pain is triggered by chewing, eating, moving his tongue, brushing his teeth, and shaving. Initially the pain was felt to be related to an infected tooth, but his pain did not improve after a root canal, and no other dental pathology was noted. He denies numbness or autonomic symptoms. He was previously taking carbamazepine 100 mg 3 times per day with clear improvement in pain, but this was associated with leukopenia and discontinued 3 weeks ago. Because the pain has been too severe to eat or drink, the patient now requires admission to the hospital for dehydration.

What do I do now?

Diagnosis

This patient's facial pain is consistent with a diagnosis of trigeminal neuralgia, currently in the setting of an acute severe exacerbation. Trigeminal neuralgia (TN) is a facial pain disorder described as recurrent severe paroxysms of pain on one side of the face, lasting from a fraction of a second to 2 minutes. The pain is described as sharp, shooting, stabbing, or electric shock–like in quality and can be triggered by maneuvers that activate the motor or sensory component of the trigeminal nerve, such as brushing the teeth, chewing/eating, talking, lightly touching the face, cool breeze on the face, shaving, or applying makeup. Patients tend to be pain-free between these shocks, though a subset of cases can develop a background more persistent pain. Even if TN tends to not be nocturnal, it can wake patients up if they touch a trigger zone in their sleep. Patients can develop a tic douloureux muscle spasm in association with pain.

When listening to this patient's story, it is important to try to identify which branches of the trigeminal nerve are being affected. This can later be relayed to radiology when ordering imaging, as well as to a surgeon or pain specialist if one is needed. Remember that the trigeminal nerve (cranial nerve V) is responsible not only for sensation of the face but also motor input to the muscles of mastication (masseter, temporalis, and pterygoids; see Table 15.1). Based on this patient's description, his pain seems to involve the right maxillary (V2) branch, predominantly.

The first step in evaluating this patient would be to perform a full neurologic examination. Secondary causes of TN, such as a mass at the cerebellopontine angle, may contribute to additional neurologic symptoms

TABLE 15.1 **Three branches of the trigeminal nerve**

Ophthalmic division (V1)	Innervates the forehead, eye, and upper eyelid
Maxillary division (V2)	Innervates the lower eyelid, cheek, upper lip, and upper gums/teeth
Mandibular division (V3)	Innervates the lower lip and chin, lower gums/teeth, and muscles of mastication (does not innervate over the angle of the jaw)

such as hearing deficit, facial weakness, or cerebellar ataxia. Therefore, particular attention should be paid to all cranial nerves, gait, and coordination. When examining facial sensation, check a small area in each division (V1, V2, V3) on each side with both light touch and pinprick to see if there is sensory deficit present. Typically, this is best checked just above the eyebrow (V1), in the mid-cheek below the eye (V2) and at the chin (V3). Check muscles of mastication by having the patient close their teeth together tightly while palpating the masseter and then the temporalis bilaterally. Some red flags on history and exam are outlined in Table 15.2. Importantly, while TN can sometimes have mild sensory changes, a dramatic reduction or loss of sensation in the distribution of the trigeminal nerve would be concerning for injury to the nerve (i.e., neuropathy) rather than neuralgia.

Trigeminal neuralgia is most commonly caused by vascular compression of the trigeminal nerve, most often by the superior cerebellar artery, but

TABLE 15.2 **Red flags on history and examination of trigeminal neuralgia**

Red flag symptom	Concerning for . . .
Numbness or persistent pain (e.g., burning, tingling, throbbing)	Trigeminal neuropathy
Systemic symptoms (e.g., fever/chills, night sweats, weight loss)	Giant cell arteritis
Only intraoral triggers (e.g., chewing, brushing teeth, touching gums)	Dental etiology such as cracked tooth, pulpitis, or abscess
Pain outside of trigeminal distribution	Alternative neuralgia such as glossopharyngeal or occipital neuralgia
Prominent autonomic symptoms (e.g., tearing, eye redness, ipsilateral rhinorrhea)	Trigeminal autonomic cephalalgia such as SUNCT*
History of erythema or rash/vesicles in region of pain	Post-herpetic neuralgia following herpes zoster
Bilateral pain or young age at onset	Alternate diagnosis or symptomatic trigeminal neuralgia

*SUNCT, short-lasting unilateral neuralgiform headache attacks with conjunctival injection and tearing

other arteries and veins may also cause neurovascular conflict. The trigeminal nerve is thought to be particularly vulnerable to compression at the *nerve root entry zone*, where it enters the pons, although compression along other parts of the trigeminal nerve also occur. When a vessel is present that is compressing, distorting, or displacing the nerve, this is referred to as *classical trigeminal neuralgia*. If the TN is related to irritation of the nerve from something other than a vessel, such as a demyelinating plaque, infarct within the brainstem, or a mass at the cerebellopontine angle, the diagnosis is referred to as *secondary trigeminal neuralgia*. If the etiology of the TN is unclear, this is referred to as *idiopathic trigeminal neuralgia*.

Work-up

Because the patient is in an acute exacerbation, it is important to consider what management options will be available to him.

This requires visualization of the trigeminal nerve. At this point, the main image to consider would be an MRI of the brain, ideally with gadolinium and high-resolution thin cuts through the posterior fossa (some facilities may refer to this as a "trigeminal nerve protocol" or something similar). This allows for not only for visualization of any neurovascular conflict along the nerve, but also evaluates for other secondary causes of TN. Because it is not uncommon for vessels to contact the trigeminal nerve in asymptomatic patients, neurovascular conflict on MRI is most compelling if there is clear evidence of compression, displacement, or atrophy ipsilateral to the pain. This patient went on to have an MRI as shown in Figure 15.1.

If the patient is more than 50 years old at the onset of pain, erythrocyte sedimentation rate (ESR) is also recommended for evaluation, to rule out giant cell arteritis mimicking TN.

If the patient has only intraoral triggers, have a low threshold for additional dental evaluation.

Treatment

First-line treatment of TN is typically pharmacologic, starting with either carbamazepine or oxcarbazepine. Patients tend to be started at low doses and gradually titrated to the lowest effective dose (see Table 15.3 for typical target dosing). Carbamazepine has the best evidence as a treatment for TN but has numerous potential side effects, such as dizziness, sedation,

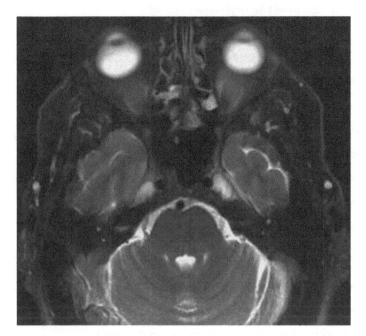

FIGURE 15.1 MRI axial T2 shows a vascular structure coursing medial to the right trigeminal nerve, displacing it laterally (white arrow).

hyponatremia, bone marrow suppression, and others. For this reason it is good practice to check a complete blood count, renal function, electrolytes, and hepatic function prior to initiation of carbamazepine and periodically thereafter. Though patients may do well on initial doses, episodic breakthrough pain may require gradual escalation of dosing over time, often to the point that the patient has difficulty tolerating the therapeutic dose. Oxcarbazepine may be better tolerated but may have a higher risk of hyponatremia.

Alternative medicines that might be helpful (based on weak evidence) include gabapentin, eslicarbazepine, baclofen, valproate, phenytoin, levetiracetam, topiramate, and botulinum toxin injections.

Typically, if the patient is unable to get control of their pain with the first medicine trial, whether due to inefficacy or intolerance, it is reasonable to consult a neurosurgeon to begin a discussion on available surgical and procedural options. This way, even if the patient chooses to try another

TABLE 15.3 **Treatment for trigeminal neuralgia**

Example preventative dosing for trigeminal neuralgia

	Starting dose	Common target dose
Carbamazepine	100 mg BID	100–300 mg QID
Oxcarbazepine	300 mg daily	600–900 mg BID
Gabapentin	300 mg daily	600–1200 mg TID
Lamotrigine	25 mg daily	100–200 mg BID
Phenytoin	100 mg TID	100–200 mg TID
Baclofen	5 mg TID	10-40 mg TID
Botulinum toxin	20–50 units, divided over trigger areas of pain	

Rescue options for trigeminal neuralgia

IV fosphenytoin (15 mg/kg over 30–60 minutes)*

IV lidocaine (5 mg/kg over 60 minutes)*

Sumatriptan, subcutaneous (3–6 mg) or nasal (20 mg)

Peripheral blocks of affected trigeminal nerve branches (using local anesthetic such as bupivacaine/lidocaine)

If available, consult neurosurgery or pain for procedural/surgical options

*Under specialist supervision with cardiac monitoring

one or two medicines, a back-up management plan is in place for refractory pain. If the patient has obvious neurovascular compression on imaging and no contraindications to surgery, often microvascular decompression is pursued first. This provides the greatest probability of relief and a long duration of effect, with approximately 64% of patients still pain-free 10 years after surgery. If there is no obvious neurovascular conflict, a neuroablative procedure (e.g., glycerol injection, balloon compression, radiofrequency thermocoagulation, stereotactic radiosurgery) would be considered. Neuroablative procedures attempt to injure the nerve to prevent the pain signal and therefore may be associated with numbness or neuropathic pain.

Similar to our patient, some patients present to urgent care settings with an acute exacerbation severe enough that they have had a difficult time eating or drinking. In this case, it is appropriate to admit the patient for hydration and rescue management of pain, while exploring procedural options with either pain medicine or neurosurgery, as available. This patient was admitted and started on IV fosphenytoin with relief of his pain. He met with neurosurgery in the hospital and was set up for an outpatient microvascular decompression.

KEY POINTS TO REMEMBER

- Not all sharp or severe unilateral facial pain is trigeminal neuralgia—it is important to differentiate from trigeminal neuropathy and other differential diagnoses.
- Due to overlapping innervation from other nerves, the best place to test sensation for each branch is just above the eyebrow (V1), in the mid-cheek below the eye, (V2) and at the chin (V3).
- If the patient is no longer able to tolerate carbamazepine or oxcarbazepine, consider a referral to neurosurgery while trying the next medicine trial. This way, a procedural plan is in place if the patient ends up refractory to medicine

Further Reading

1. Bendtsen L, Zakrzewska JM, Abbott J, et al. "European Academy of Neurology guideline on trigeminal neuralgia." *Eur J Neurol.* 2019;26(6):831–849.
2. Robertson C. "Cranial neuralgias." *Continuum* (Minneapolis). 2021;27(3):665–685. https://doi.org/10.1212/CON.0000000000000962
3. Lambru G, Zakrzewska J, Matharu M. "Trigeminal neuralgia: a practical guide." *Pract Neurol.* 2021;0:1–12. Published online first, June 2021. https://doi.org/10.1136

16 A Blow to the Head

Carolyn Bernstein

PK is a 22-year-old woman with no headache history.
She is a senior in college, avid athlete, plays soccer
in the fall and softball in the spring. She presents
to your office about 2 weeks after "heading" a ball
while playing soccer. After she impacted the ball, she
felt mildly dizzy and dazed, but has used this move
multiple times without incident. Her team won the
game, and she thought nothing more of it until 2 days
later when she realized she had a global headache,
aching in description, and mild nausea and light
sensitivity. Her mother has migraine without aura, but
PK herself has not had headaches previously. She was
so uncomfortable that she could not use her computer
for schoolwork, was having trouble concentrating,
and felt somewhat dizzy and off-balance when
walking. She sat out practice and was referred to you
for further evaluation. She denies weakness, double
vision, vomiting, or any sensory changes. PK tells you
she has no appetite and has been lying on the sofa
quietly, as music or television sounds make her feel
worse. It is hard for her to concentrate, and she feels
confused and "fuzzy." She has never experienced any

symptoms like this previously. When she describes what happened on the field, she tells you she leaned into the oncoming soccer ball, timing it carefully and twisting to propel the ball to her teammate. She does remember the force of the impact but says this was not unusual compared to previous headers.

What do I do now?

Diagnosis

PK is suffering from acute headache attributed to mild traumatic injury to the head. She did have a brief spell of dizziness and confusion right after the impact, so this would be a mild concussion. At the time, she was able to finish the game and did not report to her coach or seek further evaluation until 48 hours (about 2 days) had passed. Post-traumatic headaches are likely secondary to coup/contra-coup effects, with brain ricocheting back and forth against the skull. They are classified according to how severe the head trauma was (this would be mild; a fracture or hemorrhage would be moderate to severe) and by how long the symptoms persist. In this case, it is acute and would become a persistent headache if it lasts for more than 3 months. The majority of post-traumatic headaches that are mild do resolve within 6 months. In order to make the diagnosis, the headache must be associated with none of the following:

a. Loss of consciousness for >30 minutes
b. Glasgow Coma Scale (GCS) score <13
c. Post-traumatic amnesia lasting >24 hours[1]
d. Altered level of awareness for >24 hours
e. Imaging evidence of a traumatic head injury such as skull fracture, intracranial hemorrhage, and/or brain contusion (ICHD-3 criteria).

In addition, the patient's head injury must have been associated with one or more of the following symptoms and/or signs:

a. Transient confusion, disorientation, or impaired consciousness
b. Loss of memory for events immediately before or after the head injury
c. Two or more of the following symptoms suggestive of mild traumatic brain injury:
   i. nausea
   ii. vomiting
   iii. visual disturbances
   iv. dizziness and/or vertigo
   v. gait and/or postural imbalance
   vi. impaired memory and/or concentration.

PK meets these criteria and can be diagnosed with acute headache attributed to mild traumatic injury to the head.

Evaluation

In this case, key elements of evaluation are to ensure that nothing else is going on. She was not seen acutely; elements of the exam would likely have been consistent at that time with a normal GCS. A detailed neurologic exam must still be performed; if normal, imaging is not warranted, and the patient can be reassured that it would not change management. She is clearly dehydrated as she has been unable to keep food down, but there is no indication for laboratory testing or further diagnostic studies. The careful history and normal exam reassure you that the diagnosis is correct.

Education

Post-traumatic and post-concussive headaches may result from even minor head trauma. A typical story is from a patient who will stand up and bang their head against a shelf or piece of furniture, feel dazed for a moment, and will then develop headaches. Sports injuries can trigger, as can a mild whiplash. Often, it will take some work to tease out the inciting factor. Patients can have a variety of symptoms, and the headache can have the phenotype of migraine, tension-type headache, or be less specific. A key point is to reassure them that they will return to normal (except in rare cases) and to be patient and focus on overall wellness and rest. Classification of the headache is defined by severity of trauma and duration of symptomatology.

Management

As there are no evidence-based treatments, care of patients with post-traumatic headaches should focus on lifestyle. Treatment of post-concussive headaches is based on the primary headache phenotype it most resembles, for example, migrainous post-traumatic headaches. Rest is key, and it's important to assess sleep carefully. A lot of patients notice changes or irregularity in their sleep patterns post-concussion. Sleep hygiene and relaxation techniques before bed are important. Melatonin 3mg at the same time every evening can help, XR if difficulty staying asleep. If needed, medication to help with sleep may be useful initially, although hopefully very time-limited. Screen rest has become a component of post-concussive rehabilitation, but it's not clear that this expedites healing. The key emphasis should be on relaxing and taking a break from intensive work for a few days prior to reevaluation. This holds true for athletes and non-athletes. NSAIDs are often a good choice for pain but will not help with confusion, fatigue, or cognitive "fuzziness." Magnesium 400 mg daily, riboflavin 400 mg daily may help. Rather, hydration, good nutrition, and rest are most useful and should be emphasized. Treat nausea appropriately with medication and fluid, ginger tea. Make sure to set reasonable goals for return to work/play and to schedule follow-up visits in a timely manner. Progressive return to screen time and physical activity with frequent and short breaks is key. If the symptoms reach moderate severity with screen time or activity, a break is needed. If the symptoms don't resolve to their baseline within 45 minutes, that activity was too much, and future activity should be shorter and less intense. Integrative therapies such as craniosacral therapy have been associated with improvement from post-concussive headache, so this may be an option for patients as well.

Programs exist for both visual and vestibular rehabilitation. Focused work on balance and coordination may be extremely helpful. Visual therapies can be delivered remotely, teaching patients how to adjust their vision, reconcile quick eye movements, and decrease response to screen time. Often, optometrists will offer visual therapies, and rehabilitation centers may offer both types of work. A rehabilitation center will have the advantage of offering a multidisciplinary coordinated treatment plan. Patients ask about returning to sports; there is an increased risk of worsening symptoms with successive concussions, so this would be an important conversation to have.

KEY POINTS TO REMEMBER

- Headache and associated symptoms may follow even mild head trauma.
- All patients should be assessed in real time if possible for concussion.
- Focality in exam should prompt imaging.
- There are no medications that expedite improvement.

- Patients should be treated symptomatically.
- Focus should be on rest and self-care.
- Patients need to be reassured that they will likely improve back to baseline in a timely manner.

Further Reading

1. Mullaly W. "Concussion." *Am J Med.* 2017;130(8):885–892.
2. Langlois JA, Rutland-Brown W, Wald MM. "The epidemiology and impact of traumatic brain injury: a brief overview." *J Head Trauma Rehabil.* 2001;36:244–248.
3. Ropper AH, Gorson KC. "Clinical practice: concussion." *N Engl J Med.* 2007;356:166–172.

17 My Arteriovenous Malformation Is Clipped but My Head Still Hurts

Carolyn Bernstein

Jane is a 40-year-old woman who works as a college professor and had noted alterations in her level of consciousness ("spacing out") and forgetfulness which was unlike her baseline. She also had mild headaches that were new and different. The headache was irritating and interfered with her level of function. You evaluated her with an EEG, which showed epileptiform activity in her right temporal tip, and an MRI scan showed an arteriovenous malformation (AVM). Jane was referred to a vascular neurosurgeon who removed the AVM via a right temporal craniotomy. The surgery went smoothly, but Jane returns to your office a week later and tells you that she feels tired and has a headache. The headache is different than her pre-surgical pain; she describes a knife-like sensation along her suture line which is unremitting, causing nausea and inability to function. She has lost her appetite and tells you that she feels worse than prior to surgery.

You suggest she gives it a little more time to recover, and recommend hydration and rest. Three weeks later, she is back in your office noting ongoing pain. Again, the pain is knife-like and stabbing. She denies weakness, numbness, visual change, or vertigo. There is no photophobia or phonophobia. She is nauseated, but feels that this is from the pain. Moving around makes her feel worse. She is upset that she feels so poorly a month past her surgery.

What do I do now?

Diagnosis

Ongoing headache post-craniotomy is concerning for bleeding or infection at the wound site. Careful examination of her craniotomy site shows good healing, and there is no edema or erythema. Her neurologic exam is normal other than her ill appearance. Her complete blood count is normal, which is reassuring. Repeat imaging shows no edema or hemorrhage at the site of the AVM removal.

Once you have ruled out secondary causes, this headache fits with the diagnosis of acute headache attributed to craniotomy. To make this diagnosis, the headache must present within 7 days of the surgery and last less than 3 months (if it lasts longer, it is a persistent headache attributed to craniotomy). Patients can develop neck pain after central nervous system surgery due to positioning during the procedure, but this is different and tracks up the craniotomy site itself. The pain may trigger depression, and it is important to treat appropriately. It is not clear if the headache is secondary to sensitization of dural sensory pathways, or perhaps more peripheral due to irritation and severing of scalp musculature.

Management

Once you have reassured the patient that there is no secondary cause to the headache, focus on pain management and gentle increase in activities. NSAIDs such as ibuprofen may help, but patients may respond to a preventive therapy off-label, such as gabapentin or low-dose amitriptyline. Side effects from both of these mediations include sleepiness, which may actually be helpful in managing insomnia due to pain. Craniosacral therapy is a complementary and integrative medicine (CIM) therapy that is extremely gentle with some evidence for traumatic headaches, and this may be useful as well. Avoid vigorous massage or chiropractic treatment for these patients, but acupuncture may be another CIM therapy that helps to improve healing and decrease inflammation. Reassure your patient that the pain is very likely to resolve completely as she gets further from the surgery. Monitor for any other contributing factors such as dehydration or poor nutrition, and establish frequent communication until the headache has resolved.

KEY POINTS TO REMEMBER:

- Nearly half of patients who underwent craniotomy may develop a post-surgical headache.
- It is key to screen for other factors including hemorrhage, infection, swelling, or CSF leak.
- The headache must present within 7 days of surgery to make this diagnosis; if it lasts longer than 3 months, it is considered persistent.
- Non-prescription analgesics often help.
- Meticulous attention to lifestyle factors such as mood, sleep, and nutrition will be important.
- Gabapentin or low-dose amitriptyline may help as short-term preventive daily medications.
- There may be a role for CIM therapies as well.

Further Reading

1. Lutman B, et al. "A contemporary perspective on the management of post-craniotomy headache and pain." *Curr Pain Headache Rep.* 2018;22(10):69. https://doi.org/10.1007/s11916-018-0722-4
2. Khan S, et al. "Post procedure headache in patients treated for neurovascular arteriovenous malformations and aneurysms using endovascular therapy." *J Headache Pain.* 2016;7(1):73. https://doi.org/10.1186/s10194-016-0666-1
3. Rocha-Filho P, Sampaio A. "Post-craniotomy headache: a clinical view with a focus on the persistent form." *Headache.* 2015;55(5):733–738. https://doi.org/10.1111/head.12563

18 The Pain Persists

Chia-Chun Chiang

Jane is a 38-year old previously healthy woman
without headache history and was brought to an
emergency room with sudden-onset headache,
nausea, vertigo, and left-sided weakness. CT
angiogram of the head and neck showed dissection
of the left cervical vertebral artery, resulting in near-
complete occlusion of the left vertebral artery and
occlusion of the basilar artery (see Figure 18.1). She
received intravenous thrombolysis (tPA) and was
taken immediately for a mechanical thrombectomy,
which achieved recanalization of the basilar artery.
Brain MRI showed a left cerebellar, left-pontine, and
right occipital-lobe infarct (see Figure 18.1). She
denied history of trauma, infection, or chiropractic
manipulation. CT angiogram of the abdomen and
pelvis showed mild beading of bilateral renal arteries,
consistent with fibromuscular dysplasia. Extensive
rheumatological, autoimmune, and infectious work-up
revealed no other etiology for stroke and dissection.

Jane received anticoagulation for 3 months post-
dissection, then transitioned to aspirin 81 mg daily
without residual neurological deficits. Following the
stroke, she has experienced a debilitating headache

for around 20 days per month for the past 3 years. The headache localized mostly to the left occipital area with moderate to severe intensity and a throbbing, pressurized sensation, accompanied by photophobia, phonophobia, and nausea.

What do I do now?

Diagnosis

The International Classification of Headache Disorders (ICHD-3) describes 6.1.1 Headache attributed to ischemic stroke (cerebral infarction) as a new headache caused by an ischemic stroke and associated with neurological signs of the stroke. Development or improvement of headache should correspond to the ischemic stroke symptoms. Headaches that resolve within 3 months of the stroke are coded as 6.1.1.1 Acute Headache Attributed to Ischemic Stroke. Headaches persisting for more than 3 months are coded as 6.1.1.2 Persistent Headache Attributed to Past Ischemic Stroke. The criteria do not specify frequency. The same causation-relationship and time-window definition applies to other cerebrovascular disorder–associated headaches, including 6.5. Headache Attributed to Cervical Carotid or Vertebral Artery Disorder. In the case presented, the headache may directly correlate to the arterial dissection and is coded as 6.5.1.2 Persistent Headache or facial or neck pain attributed to past cervical carotid or vertebral artery dissection.

The incidence of post–ischemic stroke headache is between 6% and 44%. Most patients experience headache on the day of stroke with a 1- to 4-day duration. Post-stroke headache persists (>3months) in about a quarter of patients. Headache at stroke onset can be a predictor for persistent headache 6 months after stroke. Although tension-type headache is commonly reported after ischemic stroke (50%–80%), more than 50% of patients report moderate to severe pain intensity. Migraine-associated symptoms including photophobia, phonophobia, nausea, and vomiting are reported in up to 30% of patients. Risk factors for post–ischemic stroke headache include younger age (<50 years), female sex, preexisting headache disorder, larger-sized ischemic lesions, posterior (especially vertebrobasilar) circulation stroke, cortical > subcortical infarcts, and cardioembolic and large arterial atherosclerosis (rather than small-vessel disease/lacunar) infarcts.

Cervical artery dissection, either of the internal carotid artery or vertebral artery, frequently causes ischemic stroke in patients <45 years old (up to 20%). Trauma, strenuous activities, hyperextension of the neck, neck or spine manipulation, and vigorous coughing or vomiting can all precipitate dissection. Underlying connective-tissue diseases—including fibromuscular dysplasia, Ehlers–Danlos syndrome type IV, Marfan's syndrome, and other genetic vasculopathy—can predispose patients to dissection. Migraine, especially migraine without aura, correlates with higher risks of cervical artery dissection. Headache is the most frequent symptom (68%–100% of cases) of cervical artery dissection and is usually on the same side of the dissection. Migraine is a common headache phenotype, though cluster headache and thunderclap headache have been reported. Based on the location of the dissection, patients could develop symptoms including Horner's syndrome (if it involves the internal carotid artery), neurological deficits, and neck pain.

The prevalence of persistent post-cervical headache is yet to be determined. Although there have not been direct investigations comparing various headache treatments for headache after cervical artery dissection, early identification and management of headache after stroke and/or cervical artery dissection is recommended to avoid headache chronification and central sensitization.

Pathophysiology

Possible mechanisms of post-stroke headache include (1) ischemia-related disruption of the central pain modulation pathway, especially infarcts in the thalamus, brainstem, spinothalamic tract, or somatosensory cortex; (2) irritation of the intracranial pain-sensitive structures including the trigeminovascular afferents that travel along major intracranial arteries and innervate the dura; and (3) central sensitization of the nociceptive pathway.

Work-up

The first step is a thorough history and examination to evaluate for a new or change in headache pattern after the index stroke and for new neurological symptoms. Fundoscopic evaluation is crucial to rule out papilledema and secondary intracranial hypertension as a cause of the headache.

If there is a change/new headache, red flags, and/or abnormalities on neurological exam, imaging should be considered. Brain MRI is helpful to evaluate whether new infarcts or hemorrhage have occurred in the interim. Vascular imaging, including head and neck CT, or MR angiogram or conventional cerebral angiogram, can evaluate new dissections and determine whether a previous dissection has stabilized. Repeated MR or CT venogram could be considered for patients with the index stroke caused by cerebral venous sinus thrombosis or hypercoagulable state.

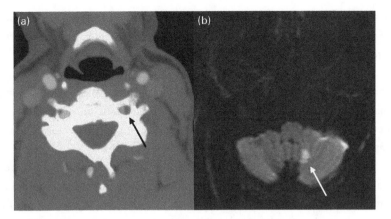

FIGURE 18.1 (A) CT angiogram showed luminal narrowing of the left vertebral artery caused by a dissection. (B) MRI showed restricted diffusion in the left cerebellum, suggesting acute ischemic infarct. Other areas of arterial occlusion and infarcts are not shown in the current figure.

Obstructive sleep apnea, depression, untreated spasticity and inadequate posture in are other common post-stroke comorbidities that can exacerbate headache and should be identified and treated.

Treatment

Headache after ischemic stroke and/or cervical artery dissection should be treated based on the headache phenotype.

Triptans and ergots should be avoided in general, due to the concern of vasoconstriction. A history of ischemic stroke is listed as a contraindication in the package inserts of the current available triptans. Acetaminophen, NSAIDs, and anti-emetics, especially those with anti-dopaminergic effect, can be used as needed to treat headache. Lasmiditan is a serotonin 5 HT-$_{1F}$ receptor agonist that received FDA approval in 2019 for the acute treatment of migraine. Available data showed that it does not cause vasoconstriction and therefore is an option for patients with a history of ischemic stroke.

Stroke is not a contraindication for calcitonin gene-related peptide (CGRP)–targeted therapy (gepants and CGRP monoclonal antibodies), but blocking CGRP, a potent vasodilator, could potentially affect the compensatory vasodilation and cerebral autoregulation if an infarct were to occur while on this therapy. Before more data become available, other vascular risk factors should be thoroughly assessed, and risks and benefits of CGRP-targeted therapy should be considered carefully, especially if the stroke is recent (≤6 months) and/or large.

Headache preventive therapy including antidepressants, beta- or calcium channel-blockers, anticonvulsants, onabotulinumtoxinA injections, nerve blocks, and neuromodulation should be chosen based on headache phenotype and other comorbidities including post-stroke depression, fatigue, central post-stroke pain, or other musculoskeletal pain.

Jane has had several follow-up MRIs and CT angiograms, which showed stable appearance of the previous infarct and healed dissection. Her blood pressure is well controlled on a beta-blocker. She takes aspirin 81 mg for stroke prevention. She has tried antidepressants and anticonvulsants without success for headache prevention. Her chronic migraine-phenotype headache that started after the stroke is currently well managed on lasmiditan as needed and onabotulinumtoxinA for prevention.

KEY POINTS TO REMEMBER

- Persistent headache attributed to past ischemic stroke and/or cervical artery dissection are common and should be identified and appropriately managed.
- Risk factors for headache associated with ischemic stroke include younger age (<50 years), female sex, preexisting headache disorder, larger size of the ischemic lesion, posterior circulation stroke, and cortical infarcts.
- Thorough evaluations, including MRI, MRA or CTA of the head and neck, MR venogram or CT venogram, fundoscopic exam, and screening for depression, limb spasticity, and obstructive sleep apnea should be considered when evaluating headache after stroke.
- For headache management, triptans and ergots should be avoided. Acetaminophen, NSAIDs, anti-emetics, and lasmiditan can be used for the acute treatment of headache. Headache-preventive therapy should be chosen according to the headache phenotype and other comorbidities. More data are needed

to evaluate the safety of CGRP-targeted therapy (gepants and CGRP monoclonal antibodies) in patients with various levels of cardiovascular/cerebrovascular risks.

Further Reading

1. Harriott AM, Karakaya F, Ayata C. "Headache after ischemic stroke: a systematic review and meta-analysis." *Neurology.* 2020;94(1):e75–e86.
2. Lai J, Harrison RA, Plecash A, Field TS. "A narrative review of persistent post-stroke headache—a new entry in the International Classification of Headache Disorders, 3rd edition." *Headache.* 2018;58(9):1442–1453.
3. Vidale S. "Headache in cervicocerebral artery dissection." *Neurol Sci.* 2020;41(Suppl 2):395–399.
4. Sheikh HU. Headache in intracranial and cervical-artery dissections. *Curr Pain Headache Rep.* 2016;20(2):8.

19 Catch It Before It Bursts: Headache and Posterior Communicating Artery Aneurysm

Deena E. Kuruvilla

KAS, a 52-year-old woman with a history of hypertension, tobacco use, migraine without aura, and migraine with aura presents to your clinic with a severe new headache for 2 weeks which has not been alleviated by sumatriptan, rizatriptan, eletriptan, a course of nonsteroidal anti-inflammatory medication, and a course of rimegepant. The patient reports that she has her typical migraine pain as well as this new type of headache. She reports her typical migraine pain is continuous and daily at a baseline level of 2/10 with exacerbations to a 6/10 once a week. She describes her typical migraine as holocranial throbbing associated with photophobia, phonophobia, nausea, and vomiting, usually preceded by flashing lights and wavy lines. Her new headache she describes as a sudden-onset, sharp pain in the left frontal lobe that only occurs with exercise, coughing, and bowel movements. She describes this pain as a 9–10/10 when it occurs, and lasts until she stops exerting herself. She denies a positional component, focal weakness, focal numbness, and speech changes with this new headache. On the physical exam, her blood pressure is elevated to 189/101, pulse is 101, and temperature is 98. Her cranial nerve exam shows a left ptosis. Her left pupil is 5 mm, dilated and sluggish. Her right pupil is 2.5 mm and reactive. She has intact extraocular movements and the rest of her neurological exam is unrevealing.

What do I do now?

brupt changes in the patient's baseline headache frequency or severity warrant urgent evaluation. Changes on the patient's neurological exam warrant urgent evaluation. There are multiple red flags in this case, including her elevated blood pressure, which should prompt you to send this patient to the emergency department (ED). This patient needs neuroimaging, and she needs it now!

Headache is the fifth most common chief complaint among patients in the ED. Identifying red flags or danger signs in a patient's history is critical for the identification of a secondary cause for headache. A mnemonic was developed by Dodick et al. to assist with identifying danger signs called SNOOP4. A sudden-onset headache, also known as a thunderclap headache (TCH), should prompt one to consider vascular etiologies. Vascular etiologies for TCH include subarachnoid hemorrhage (SAH), acute stroke, reversible cerebral vasoconstriction syndrome (RCVS), cerebral venous sinus thrombosis (CVT), arterial dissection, posterior reversible encephalopathy syndrome (PRES), pituitary apoplexy, and unruptured intracranial aneurysm. Non-vascular causes to consider include colloid cyst, infection, sphenoid sinusitis, and intracranial hypotension.

Plain computerized tomography scan (CT scan) can be used to rapidly assess the brain and detect any signs of intracranial hemorrhage. Contrast-enhanced computerized tomography angiography (CTA) of the head and neck can also rapidly identify vascular malformations such as aneurysm, dissection, or arterial narrowing followed by dilation as seen in RCVS. Magnetic resonance imaging (MRI) and magnetic resonance angiography (MRA) are also ideal approaches to identifying secondary causes for headache. There are pros and cons when deciding which to order. CT scan is faster than MRI, and therefore is more useful with trauma and or other neurological emergencies. CT scan is more cost effective than MRI and can be used in patients with implantable medical devices such as pacemakers and stimulators. MRI does not use ionizing radiation and may be preferred over CT in children or other patients who should have limited radiation exposure. MRI outlines the brain anatomy in more detail and is therefore more sensitive and specific for lesions in the brain. To identify acute hemorrhage, bone fracture, or other neurological emergency, a CT scan without contrast should be ordered for this patient KAS, followed by a CTA head and neck with contrast to identify a vascular abnormality.

A CTA of the head and neck for our patient KAS revealed a left posterior communicating artery aneurysm (PCoA), which had not ruptured. This study as well as a CT scan of the head revealed no evidence of a rupture or SAH. The patient was taken for a cerebral angiography, which is the gold standard for the diagnosis of intracranial aneurysms. The neurosurgery team identified the aneurysm, and she was successfully treated with endovascular coiling.

PCoAs account for 45.9% of all aneurysms, and due to the high risk of morbidity and mortality, the diagnosis should not be delayed. PCoAs are more likely to rupture than other types of aneurysms. PCoAs arise from the internal carotid artery (ICA) and are anatomically next to the oculomotor nerve. On neurological exam, partial or complete oculomotor nerve palsy (ONP) occurs in 30%–50% of people with PCoA. Interventional treatment approaches include microsurgical clipping, or endovascular approaches such as primary coiling, stent-assisted coiling, or dual catheter techniques. A study suggests that patients receiving surgical clipping had a higher full recovery rate compared to patients who received endovascular approaches. It is important to counsel patients regarding smoking cessation, because studies have shown that smoking is the single greatest risk factor which contributes to aneurysm growth and subsequent rupture. Other factors include aneurysm size, age, female gender, and hypertension. Complications of PCoAs include rupture with SAH, intraparenchymal hemorrhage (IPH), non-traumatic subdural hematoma (SDH), and persistent ONP and other significant neurological disability.

When treating headache in patients with PCoAs, NSAIDs should be avoided, as they increase the bleeding risk, and triptans should be used with caution during the periprocedural period, as they have vasoconstrictive effects. There is no evidence thus far that triptans are contraindicated in unruptured cerebral aneurysms. Oral acetaminophen, intravenous or oral metoclopramide, intravenous or oral prochlorperazine, intravenous caffeine, and intranasal lidocaine are evidence-based options to consider in these patients.

- A sudden change in headache frequency or severity, or change in the quality of baseline headaches warrants an urgent evaluation.
- An abnormal neurological exam should prompt urgent neuroimaging.
- Thunderclap headache is a warning sign for several non-vascular and vascular etiologies for headache.
- Posterior communicating artery aneurysms carry a very high risk of rupture and subsequent morbidity and mortality.
- Prompt consultation with a neurosurgeon or interventional neuroradiologist when evaluating intracranial aneurysms is critical.

Acknowledgment: Diya Girish Kumar, Medical Intern, Westport Headache Institute

Further Reading

1. Stovner LJ, Hagen K, Jensen R, et al. "The global burden of headache: a documentation of headache prevalence and disability worldwide." *Cephalalgia* 2007;27:193–210. doi:10.1111/j.1468-2982.2007.01288.x

2. Dodick DW. "Diagnosing secondary and primary headache disorders." *Continuum.* 2021;27:572–585.

3. Khan M, et al. "Multidisciplinary headache clinic—a new model for headache care." *J Neurol. Sci* 2019;405(Suppl):70.

4. Sullivan MG. "Acronym helps identify red flags in acute severe headache." *Int Med News.* 2006;39:31.

5. McCaig LF, Burt CW. *National Hospital Ambulatory Medical Care Survey: 2003 Emergency Department Summary.* (2005).

6. Dodick D. "Pearls: headache." *Sem Neurol.* 2010;30:074–081.

7. Ravishankar K. "WHICH headache to investigate, WHEN, and HOW?" *Headache.* 2016;56:1685–1697.

8. Guo S, Wu X. "An unruptured posterior communicating artery aneurysm ruptured during angiography: a case report." *Medicine.* 2019;**98**:e17785.

9. Mandell DM, et al. "Intracranial vessel wall MRI: principles and expert consensus recommendations of the American Society of Neuroradiology." *Am J Neuroradiol.* 2017;38:218–229.

10. Masdeu JC, Gadhia R, Faridar A. "Brain CT and MRI." *Handbook of Clinical Neurology.* 2016:1037–1054. https://doi.org/10.1016/b978-0-444-53486-6.00054-5

11. Bruneton JN. "Practical differential diagnosis for CT and MRI." *Clin Imaging.* 2009;33:76.

12. Salmon E, Bernard Ir. C, Hustinx R. "Pitfalls and limitations of PET/CT in brain imaging. *Semin Nucl Med.* 2015;45:541–551.

13. Bhatkar S, et al. "Magnetic resonance imaging (MRI) versus computed tomographic scan (CT scan) of brain in evaluation of suspected cavernous sinus syndrome." *Neuroradiol J.* 2020;33:501–507.

14. Liu J, et al. "Treatment of true posterior communicating artery aneurysms: Endovascular experience in a single center." *Interv Neuroradiol.* 2020;26:55–60.

15. Zimmer DV. "Oculomotor nerve palsy from posterior communicating artery aneurysm." *J La State Med Soc.* 1991;143:22–25.

16. Tominari S, et al. "Prediction model for 3-year rupture risk of unruptured cerebral aneurysms in Japanese patients." *Ann Neurol.* 2015;77:1050–1059.

17. Forget TR Jr, et al. "A review of size and location of ruptured intracranial aneurysms." *Neurosurgery.* 2001;49:1322–1325; discussion 1325–6.

18. Corliss BM, Hoh BL. "Posterior communicating artery aneurysm presenting with and without third nerve palsy." *Cerebrovasc Neurosurg.* 2019:15–24. https://doi.org/10.1093/med/9780190887728.003.0003

19. Tian L-Q, Fu Q-X. "Recovery of posterior communicating artery aneurysm induced oculomotor nerve palsy: a comparison between surgical clipping and endovascular embolization." *BMC Neurol.* 2020;20:351.

20. Juvela S. "Natural history of unruptured intracranial aneurysms: risks for aneurysm formation, growth, and rupture." *Acta Neurochir Suppl.* 2002;82:27–30.

21. Juvela S, Porras M, Poussa K. "Natural history of unruptured intracranial aneurysms: probability of and risk factors for aneurysm rupture." *J Neurosurgery.* 2008;108:1052–1060.

22. Donauer E, et al. "Posterior communicating artery aneurysm: subarachnoid hemorrhage from a small aneurysm located on an infundibulum of the posterior communicating artery; partial clipping of the aneurysm, followed by endovascular flow diversion, with good clinical outcome." *The Aneurysm Casebook* 2019:1–13. https://doi.org/10.1007/978-3-319-70267-4_96-1

23. Baron EP. "Headache, cerebral aneurysms, and the use of triptans and ergot derivatives." *Headache.* 2015;55:739–747.

24. Gilmore B, Michael M. "Treatment of acute migraine headache." *Am Fam Physician.* 2011;83:271–280.

20 "Itis" Means There Is Inflammation Somewhere . . .

Yulia Orlova and Bryce Buchowicz

A 74-year-old white Caucasian woman presents
with a new throbbing headache for 2 weeks in the
right temporal area which is tender to touch. It is
aggravated by talking and chewing, with a brief
episode of vision loss and blurry vision in her
right eye and low-grade fever. She has an elevated
ESR of 86 mm/hr and CRP of 24 mg/L. CBC shows
hemoglobin of 9.1 g/dL and thrombocytosis with
platelet level of 550,000. Temporal artery biopsy of the
right temporal artery was negative. Ultrasound of the
right temporal artery revealed a "halo" sign.

What do I do now?

A new onset of headache associated with jaw claudication and transient visual loss in this older woman is highly suspicious for giant cell arteritis.

Giant cell arteritis (GCA) is a chronic systemic vasculitis of large and medium size arteries characterized by granulomatous inflammation leading to segmental luminal narrowing. GCA is a medical emergency because of the risk of permanent visual loss (8%–30%) and risk of stroke (3%–7%). GCA is the most common vasculitis that affects people ≥50 and older, with the highest incidence in the eighth decade of life. The largest prevalence of GCA is seen in people of Northern European ancestry with incidence 15 to 25 cases per 100,000 persons over 50 years of age.

GCA represents a spectrum of overlapping conditions that includes cranial GCA, extracranial or large-vessel GCA, and polymyalgia rheumatica (PMR).

Release of cytokines from an inflammatory state leads to nonspecific constitutional symptoms such as malaise, fatigue, low-grade fever that can be accompanied by anemia, and elevated acute-phase reactants such as ESR, CRP, and thrombocytosis. PMR symptoms include aching and morning stiffness in the neck, shoulder, and pelvic girdle, accompanied by elevated inflammatory markers.

Specific local findings of GCA reflect ischemic complications from arteritis. Cranial GCA most commonly affects extracranial arteries such as temporal, ophthalmic, and posterior ciliary arteries. Large-vessel GCA is an extracranial form that affects large supra-aortic arteries and/or the aorta.

New onset of headache in an individual older than 60 years is reported in more than two-thirds of patients with GCA. This can raise the suspicion of GCA and prompt appropriate investigation, but as an isolated symptom it has low diagnostic value.

Headache in GCA can have various patterns. It has no specific features and can be constant or intermittent, and in any location with various intensities. It can mimic tension-type headache, migraine, cluster headache, or even occipital neuralgia when the occipital artery is involved. Occipito-nuchal pain can also be a nonspecific sign of truncal pain from polymyalgia rheumatica. Facial pain from facial artery vasculitis can be mistaken for trigeminal neuralgia.

Ophthalmic signs and symptoms are seen in up to 30% of patients with GCA and include anterior ischemic optic neuropathy, central retinal artery occlusion, branch retinal artery occlusion, posterior ischemic optic neuropathy, and choroidal infarction that can lead to persistent visual loss, with or without amaurosis fugax. Isolated or multiple oculomotor cranial nerve palsies from ischemic neuropathy can lead to transient or persistent diplopia. Occipital infarction can also cause persistent visual loss.

Jaw claudication is seen in about 50% of patients with GCA, presenting as weakness and jaw discomfort with chewing hard food and prolonged talking. Less common ischemic complications include tongue claudication with tongue weakness, paresthesias, and pain that can result in tongue necrosis.

Patients with extracranial disease are less likely to have headache and visual loss, but can have limb claudication, Raynaud's phenomenon, aortitis, and thoracic and abdominal aneurysms.

Diagnosis of GCA requires detailed clinical history, thorough evaluation, and additional tests. There are no universally accepted diagnostic criteria. 1990 American College of Rheumatology (ACR) criteria for GCA were designed as classification criteria to differentiate from other forms of vasculitis but have been frequently misused for diagnosis of this disease.

Several tools are proposed to aid in diagnosis of GCA. Revised ACR criteria for early diagnosis of GCA (2016) offers a scoring system that can aid in stratifying patients who need a temporal artery biopsy. GCA risk calculator is another tool available online to assess pre-test probability of this condition and includes age, gender, new headache, temporal artery tenderness or decreased pulse, jaw or tongue claudication, vision loss (AION, PION, CRAO), diplopia, ESR, CRP, and platelets count (available at https://goo.gl/THCnuU). Although inflammatory markers such as ESR, CRP, and elevated platelets count are not specific for GCA and can be normal in up to 10% of patients, they can be useful to monitor for activity of the disease.

Presence of symptoms of arterial ischemia (jaw claudication, transient visual loss) and systemic inflammation (low-grade fever, anemia, thrombocytosis, elevated ESR and CRP) in our case raises the suspicion for GCA, but a confirmatory diagnostic test is required.

Confirmatory tests include either temporal artery biopsy at least 1 cm in length, preferably 2–3 cm, or an ultrasound of the temporal and axillary arteries, or both. Ultrasonography can detect a sign of inflammation of the vessel wall with a "halo sign," a non-compressible hypoechoic ring around the artery lumen. Magnetic resonance imaging (MRI) with MR angiogram (MRA) can also visualize temporal arteries and demonstrate wall artery edema when used with contrast, but is limited due to the cost and need for contrast.

Temporal artery biopsy (TAB) is considered a "gold standard" for diagnosis of cranial GCA, although it may not be easily available, and interpretation may not be straightforward. Sensitivity of TAB is estimated 60%–70%, compatible with ultrasonography and MRI of temporal arteries. To increase the diagnostic value of artery biopsy, the most symptomatic artery should be selected for biopsy, but bilateral temporal artery biopsies have low value.

Histopathological findings of GCA include panarteritis, usually most pronounced in the media. Fragmentation of internal elastic membrane and presence of CD4+ lymphocytes and macrophages are signs of active arteritis, but presence of giant cells is not required for diagnosis. GCA is a non-necrotizing vasculitis, and presence of fibrinoid necrosis should prompt an alternative diagnosis, particularly granulomatosis with polyangiitis and polyarteritis nodosa (PAN) that may involve cranial arteries but requires different treatment.

TAB in our case was negative, which posed a diagnostic challenge. Limited sensitivity of TAB is often attributed to skip lesions, corticosteroid therapy prior to biopsy, or sparing of temporal arteries, especially when large vessels are involved. However, when the temporal artery segment (2–3 cm) is collected by an experienced surgeon, skip lesions have only a minor impact on negative results of biopsy. Steroid therapy for up to 2 weeks has little effect on positive rate.

Temporal arteries can be spared in large-vessel GCA, and 30%–40% of patients with this form have negative TAB results. When large-vessel disease is suspected, advanced vascular imaging might be necessary, including MRA, computed tomography angiography (CTA), or positron emission tomography with 2-deoxy-2-[fluorine-18] fluoro- D-glucose integrated with computed tomography (^{18}F-FDG PET/CT), although CT studies pose additional risk of exposure to radiation, and PET has limited availability.

In our case, ultrasound of the temporal artery revealed hypoechoic wall thickening ("halo" sign), which is supportive for diagnosis of vasculitis, despite negative results of TAB.

Once GCA is suspected, immediate corticosteroid therapy should be initiated while work-up is commencing. Steroid treatment should not be delayed for temporal artery biopsy; however, acute-phase reactants should be drawn prior to steroid treatment.

A typical initial dose of oral corticosteroids is 40 to 60 mg of prednisone daily. For those with cranial ischemic symptoms, such as visual symptoms or stroke, 3-day induction with IV methylprednisolone at 1g per day followed by oral taper starting at 1 mg/kg/day (maximum 60 mg per day) is recommended. Once vision loss has occurred, it is often permanent. Treatment is focused on prevention of vision loss in the contralateral eye, as untreated GCA vasculitis can cause bilateral blindness in days to a week.

High doses of oral steroids are continued until there is a resolution of clinical symptoms and normalization of inflammatory markers. A very slow steroid taper (5 mg or less per week) is advised, with increase in dose if symptoms return. Corticosteroids are used for 12 to 18 months, or even longer, depending on clinical response.

The majority of patients develop corticosteroid-induced side effects including posterior subcapsular cataracts, osteonecrosis, vertebral compression fractures, infection, diabetes mellitus, peptic ulcer, hypertension, and neuropsychiatric effects including depression. Proton pump inhibitors for gastrointestinal protection, supplemental calcium and vitamin D, and bone-sparing treatment such as bisphosphonates should be considered in patients who are taking high doses of corticosteroids.

Although most patients have significant clinical improvement within 24–48 hours of therapy, relapse occurs in up to two-thirds of patients. In those with protracted steroid therapy due to relapses and those at high risk for steroid toxicity, adjunctive steroid-sparing agents such as methotrexate (MTX) and tocilizumab (TCZ) should be considered. Other conventional immunosuppressants are not effective.

MTX at dose 7.5–15 mg per week was helpful in reducing the duration of steroid therapy, but the effect was modest.

Tocilizumab (TCZ), IL-6 receptor inhibitor, can be administered intravenously at the dose 4–8 mg/kg every 4 weeks, or subcutaneously at a dose

162 mg every week or every other week in combination with a tapering dose of corticosteroids, and continued as monotherapy after the discontinuation of corticosteroids. Side effects include transient neutropenia, elevation of triglycerides, and abnormal liver function tests. Patients treated with TCZ had higher risk of gastrointestinal perforation, and it is contraindicated in patients with diverticular disease. Because acute-phase response is suppressed during the therapy with TCZ, disease activity may be difficult to assess, which might require vascular imaging during the follow-up.

PEARLS

- New onset of headache in an individual older than 60 should raise the suspicion for GCA but is not sufficient to establish diagnosis.
- Patients with suspected GCA should have confirmatory tests: either a temporal artery biopsy at least 1 cm in length, or an ultrasound of the temporal and axillary arteries, or both.
- Temporal artery biopsy is most valuable when performed within 2 weeks from initiation of steroid therapy.
- High dose of corticosteroids is the most effective treatment of GCA and should be initiated early.
- Consider steroid-sparing therapy in patients at risk for side effects from corticosteroid therapy and those with relapses despite adequate corticosteroid therapy.

Further Reading
1. Mollan SP, Paemeleire K, Versijpt J, Luqmani R, Sinclair AJ. "European Headache Federation recommendations for neurologists managing giant cell arteritis." *J Headache Pain*. 2020;21:28.
2. Lyons HS, Quick V, Sinclair AJ, Nagaraju S, Mollan SP. "A new era for giant cell arteritis." *Eye*. 2020;34:1013–1026.
3. Levin M, Ward TN. "Horton's disease: past and present." *Curr Pain Headache Rep.* 2005;9:259–263.

21 Recurrent Thunderclap Headache

Sandhya Mehla

Joe is a 24-year-old man with a history of depression and episodic migraine without aura (headache frequency of 2 days per year), and presents to the headache clinic for a new-onset thunderclap headache. Headache started while taking a shower, 10 days prior to the visit, and has been daily continuous since onset. Headache is bilateral occipital and frontotemporal, severity ranging from 3/10 to 10/10, which worsens to peak within seconds upon straining and is associated with severe nausea, photophobia, and significant vertigo since onset but without any other neurological symptoms. Patient denies pulsatile tinnitus, but any change in position worsens the severity of headache. He has been taking Tramadol with some relief. There is no family history of migraine, intracranial aneurysm, or intracranial hemorrhage. He smokes marijuana every day. For medications, he is on escitalopram 15 mg and Claritin every day, and Tramadol as needed since the headache onset. On review of systems, he lost 15 pounds in 10 days because of severe nausea and headache, and he has chronic nasal congestion.

His exam is unremarkable for any focal neurological deficits, but he has significant myalgia in trapezius muscles bilaterally and cranial allodynia bilaterally. A non-contrast head CT (NCHCT) performed on day 1 in the emergency department was unremarkable. He did not have any viral infection prior to this headache.

What do I do now?

DIAGNOSIS

Contrary to common belief, a thunderclap headache is a headache that reaches maximum intensity within seconds of onset (not necessarily the worst headache of life). Joe presents with two red flags, which are concerning for a secondary headache: new headache different from his prior migraine attacks, and thunderclap onset. The differential diagnosis includes subarachnoid hemorrhage (SAH), reversible cerebral vasoconstriction syndrome (RCVS), cerebral venous sinus thrombosis (CVST), intracerebral hemorrhage (ICH), arterial dissection, pituitary apoplexy, third ventricle colloid cyst, and pheochromocytoma. The unremarkable NCHCT places SAH, ICH, and colloid cyst lower on the differential. RCVS is higher on the differential given the recurrent character of his thunderclap headache and exposure to vasoactive substances. CSVT is also high on the differential given the persistent nature of his headache.

RCVS encompasses multiple different conditions that all lead to a fully reversible constriction of cerebral blood vessels. These conditions include Call Fleming syndrome, postpartum angiopathy, drug-induced arteriopathy, and migraine-related vasospasm. Although commonly considered a benign disorder, serious complications can occur. RCVS is more common in women than men, with highest age prevalence in the 40s. Clinically, RCVS can be very heterogeneous, but more than 90% of patients present with recurrent thunderclap headache. Nearly 70% of patients with RCVS have a trigger, most commonly a vasoactive agent. RCVS can occur both with the first-time or long-standing use of serotonergic or adrenergic agents. Various triggers for RCVS are listed in Box 21.1. The pathophysiology of RCVS is believed to be a disturbance in the autoregulation of vessel tone. RCVS may be on the spectrum of posterior reversible encephalopathy syndrome (PRES).

Work-up

The first step in the evaluation of an acute thunderclap headache is to rule out a SAH or ICH with a **NCHCT**. The sensitivity of NCHCT for SAH is 98% within the first 12 hours of the ictus and 93% within 24 hours. If the imaging is negative but there is a clinical suspicion, a **lumbar puncture** must be done to look for xanthochromia with a spectrophotometry.

It has 90% sensitivity for SAH after 12 hours of symptom onset. Joe's cerebrospinal fluid (CSF) analysis is unremarkable, and there is no xanthochromia.

If the NCHCT and CSF analysis are unremarkable, the next step is obtaining **vessel imaging,** either via computed tomography angiogram (CTA) or non-contrast magnetic resonance angiogram (MRA) of the head and neck. MRA has about 80% sensitivity in identifying RCVS-related vasospasm. However, peak vasospasm occurs between 2 to 3 weeks of onset. Therefore, if the initial vessel imaging is normal and the suspicion for RCVS is high because of recurrent thunderclap headache or presence of triggers, the vessel imaging should be repeated 2 weeks later. Although not readily available at all centers, transcranial dopplers can also be used to detect vasospasm; however, sensitivity is based on the temporal window.

Given the persistent character of his headaches and concern for CSVT, an MRV was also obtained for Joe, which was unremarkable. Urine toxicology screens should be performed for vasoactive substance exposure.

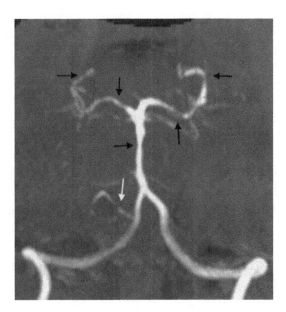

FIGURE 21.1 MRA head showing bilateral vertebral artery (VA), basilar artery, bilateral posterior cerebral arteries (PCA) and right posterior inferior cerebellar artery (PICA). Black arrows point to the areas of stenoses in basilar artery and bilateral PCAs. White arrow points to stenosis in the right PICA.

In Joe's case, the MRA of the head showed diffuse segmental vasocon-striction in the posterior circulation (see Figure 21.1). Because of the seg-mental vasoconstriction on imaging, vasculitis/angiitis is now considered higher on differential diagnosis. The RCVS2 clinical score helps distin-guish RCVS from other arteriopathies. The key variables of the RCVS2 that have the highest specificity for RCVS are recurrent thunderclap head-ache, presence of trigger with normal imaging, and convexal SAH. A brain MRI is obtained, which in Joe's case is unremarkable. Joe's RCVS2 score is 8. Almost all patients with primary angiitis of the central nervous system (PACNS) have abnormal MRI brain compared to only 30% with RCVS. Early MRI findings of RCVS include edema on the FLAIR, hyperintensity on ADC, and hyperintense vessel sign. Given the concern for angiitis in this case, a cerebral angiogram is performed and unremarkable. When con-cerned for vasculitis/angiitis, further blood analysis should be done to eval-uate for secondary etiologies.

Management

A major step in treatment is discontinuing all vasoactive medications or other pharmacological agents which can potentially trigger vasospasm. In this case, Joe was asked to completely stop smoking marijuana and taking escitalopram.

Calcium channel blockers (CCBs) are effective in reducing the headache but do not help the prognosis. Nimodipine is commonly used in inpatient settings; however, verapamil is the drug of choice in outpatient settings. Longer-acting formulation of verapamil is commonly used for better compliance at a starting dose of 120 mg daily, and can be increased to 120 mg twice a day based on clinical response. If a higher dose is required, electrocardiogram monitoring should be performed, as CCBs can cause atrioventricular nodal block. This use of CCBs is based on clinical expertise; clinical trials are lacking. Joe's headache quickly improved with long-acting verapamil 120 mg daily.

Prognosis

An early follow-up is recommended, as 14% of patients get readmitted for ongoing or recurrent RCVS symptoms. Of note, risk factors for relapse include a history of migraine and exercise/exertion as triggers. Vasoconstriction in RCVS typically resolves in 3 months.

Complications of RCVS include seizures, transient focal neurological deficits, cerebral infarcts that mainly occur in watershed areas, convexal SAH, intraparenchymal hemorrhage, and cerebral edema. Transient focal neurological deficits can be similar to transient ischemic attacks but can mimic migraine aura as well. Cerebral edema is typically noted in distribution similar to what is seen in PRES. In severe cases with rapidly progressing neurological symptoms, catheter angiogram with intra-arterial vasodilator treatment has some role in management of RCVS, but there is a concern about reperfusion injury.

Post-RCVS headache occurs in about 50% of the patients and usually has migrainous features. Of the patients with post-RCVS headache, 10% have disability from it and at least 5% have a RCVS recurrence.

Joe remains headache free at his 1-month, 3-month, and 6-month follow-ups, with no recurrence of thunderclap headache. On the 3-month follow-up MRA head, the vasoconstriction is significantly improved but persists in some areas. He continues to take verapamil. There is a risk benefit discussion regarding restarting a serotonin and norepinephrine reuptake inhibitor (SNRI), as he has depression. Joe opts for behavioral therapy instead of pharmacological management, which is effective. If using a pharmacological agent is absolutely needed, non-serotonergic agents can be considered.

PEARLS OF WISDOM AND CAUTIONARY STEPS

1. In recurrent TCH with normal initial diagnostic imaging (NCHCT + vessel imaging), consider repeating vessel imaging and trigger search before making the diagnosis of primary thunderclap headache.
2. Recurrent TCH, presence of triggers with normal brain imaging, and convexal SAH are the biggest predictors of RCVS.
3. Discontinue all the vasoactive and triggering medications immediately upon suspicion of RCVS.
4. RCVS may not always be a benign syndrome. Complications like SAH, ischemic stroke, and cerebral edema can occur.
5. Calcium channel blockers provide symptomatic relief in headache but do not improve prognosis.
6. Follow-up imaging at 3 months is important, as the reversible nature of the vasoconstriction is key to the diagnosis.

Further Reading

1. Ducros A. "Reversible cerebral vasoconstriction syndrome." *Lancet Neurol.* 2012;11:906–917.
2. Ducros A, Wolff V. "The typical thunderclap headache of reversible cerebral vasoconstriction syndrome and its various triggers." *Headache.* 2016;56(4):657–673. https://doi.org/10.1111/head.12797
3. Rocha EA, Topcuoglu MA, Silva GS, Singhal AB. "RCVS2 score and diagnostic approach for reversible cerebral vasoconstriction syndrome." *Neurology.* 2019;92(7):e639–e647. https://doi.org/10.1212/WNL.0000000000006917

22 A Question of Headache and Hemorrhage

Huma U. Sheikh

A 67-year-old woman with a history of mild cognitive impairment, who has recently moved in with her daughter, complains of a headache in the back of her head, starting during breakfast. She does not note a history of headaches when she was younger, but did note a severe headache about 5 months ago, for which she did not seek help and that resolved over a week. Her daughter noted that she may have had some slurring of speech during that time but was not sure. Her daughter notes that her mother has begun to forget dates and has some difficulty with her morning routine in the last few weeks. On exam, the patient has a right facial droop, mild right-sided weakness in the arm with a pronator drift in the arm and leg. She has trouble naming objects but can follow all commands and has fluent speech. An initial CT scan showed a 3 cc area of intracerebral hemorrhage in the left medial temporal lobe. Atrial fibrillation (AF) is found on routine telemetry monitoring.

What do I do now?

Headache Red Flags

There are some important points highlighted in this case. The first area to focus on is the management of headaches in the older population. Headache is a common presenting symptom in the emergency room. The most common underlying etiology is a primary headache syndrome, of which migraine is the most common. However, it is important to be aware of red flags when someone presents with a headache. This patient has concerning factors, including onset in an older age, headache that is acute and severe at onset, as well as a headache with other neurological signs. A headache that comes on acutely and becomes severe over seconds or minutes is also concerning. In this case, the intracerebral hemorrhage is likely the cause of her headache. The prior history of an acute headache may have also been a previous secondary issue. This would alert you to a possibility of previous hemorrhage and therefore may heighten your concern for etiologies where there may be repeated hemorrhages.

Differential for Intracerebral Hemorrhage (ICH)

The other important point in this case is the differential for intracerebral hemorrhage. The two largest etiologies include hypertensive hemorrhage and cerebral amyloid angiopathy (CAA). Other less frequent causes include arteriovenous malformation, cavernous angiomas, hemorrhagic metastasis, and aneurysmal rupture, in addition to others. The location can be helpful in narrowing the differential, and imaging, including magnetic resonance imaging (MRI) along with magnetic resonance angiogram (MRA) of the intracerebral vasculature with contrast is usually done to look for an underlying lesion.

In this case, the location of this acute hemorrhage, along with evidence of previous hemorrhage on gradient ECHO images of MRI, in addition to the history of MCI should alert one to the possibility of CAA.

CEREBRAL AMYLOID ANGIOPATHY

Cerebral amyloid angiopathy refers to a condition where there are amyloid-Beta deposits in the cerebrovasculature. It is now recognized as a major contributor to intracerebral hemorrhage and has been identified as a contributing factor to cognitive decline. Although there is a link to Alzheimer's disease, these are two clinically different conditions in terms of pathophysiology. The pathological hallmarks of CAA include involvement of small arterioles and capillaries of the leptomeninges and cerebral cortex; distribution in the posterior lobar regions, associated with increased age and dementia; and the observation that white matter small vessels are not involved. There is also not a clear association with other cardiovascular risk factors like hypertension and atherosclerosis, nor is there any clear link to systemic amyloidosis.

Autopsy studies show that CAA is present in about 20%–40% of patients not known to have dementia, and that rate increases to about 50%–60% in elderly patients with dementia. These rates are much higher in those with Alzheimer's, where the rates can be as high as 85%–95%. CAA is thought to be a contributing factor in about 12%–20% of intracerebral hemorrhages. Definitive diagnosis is made through histopathologic confirmation; however, imaging is usually helpful in raising the suspicion. MRI findings typically include multiple cortical micro-hemorrhages on gradient echo, especially in patients over the age of 55.

The clinical presentation of CAA includes intracerebral hemorrhage that is classically in lobar distribution and spontaneous, along with cognitive impairment or frank dementia. These patients may also have transient focal spells that are linked to episodes of bleeding.

To Anticoagulate or Not Anticoagulate: That Is the Question

One other decision in this patient is whether or not to start anticoagulation, since she is now at high risk of stroke given her AF. This involves balancing the risk of ischemic stroke due to atrial fibrillation (AF) versus the risk of recurrent hemorrhage due to CAA. The chances of having both CAA and AF increase as the population ages, although CAA is not always detected unless there is adequate imaging. In deciding whether or not to start anticoagulation, there are other criteria that are used, including the overall risk of ischemic stroke. The risk of stroke in those with AF is increased with the presence of other factors, including diabetes mellitus, previous stroke and hypertension, as well as age. In cases of previous hemorrhage, using anticoagulation for AF is risky, especially if there are more lobar hemorrhages.

However, to date there are no clear guidelines on the use of anticoagulation in AF after previous intracerebral hemorrhage secondary to CAA. In cases that are deemed risky, it can be helpful to discuss possible other options including percutaneously implanted closure devices that block off the left atrial appendage, the area most thought to develop clots that can then travel to the brain. Further studies are needed to determine its safety and validity. These cases are often challenging and require an individualized approach.

KEY POINTS TO REMEMBER

- CAA may present with migraine aura-like transient focal neurological episodes (TFNE) or with a headache with red flags (older age of onset, thunderclap, with neurological focal deficits, for example).
- Consider cerebral amyloid angiopathy in patients who are older with a history of dementia and present with intracerebral hemorrhage.
- GRE sequencing on MRI can be a helpful tool to determine if there is high probability of CAA.
- Risk of bleeding should be taken into consideration when deciding on anti-platelet use or anticoagulation.

Further Reading
1. Do TP, Remmers A, et al. "Red and orange flags for secondary headaches in clinical practice." *Neurology.* 2019;92(3):134–144.
2. Yeh SJ, Tang SC, Tsai LK, Jeng JS. "Pathogenetical subtypes of recurrent intracerebral hemorrhage: designations by SMASH-U classification system." *Stroke.* 2014;45:2636–2642.
3. Meretoja A, Strbian D, Putaala J, Curtze S, Haapaniemi E, Mustanoja S, et al. "SMASH-U: a proposal for etiologic classification of intracerebral hemorrhage." *Stroke.* 2012;43:2592–2597.
4. Yamada M, Tsukagoshi H, Otomo E, Hayakawa M. "Cerebral amyloid angiopathy in the aged." *J Neurol.* 1987;234:371–376.
5. Charidimou A, Boulouis G, Gurol ME, et al. « Emerging concepts in sporadic cerebral amyloid angiopathy." *Brain.* 2017;140(7):1829–1850.
6. Yamada M. "Cerebral amyloid angiopathy: emerging concepts." *J Stroke.* 2015;17:17–30.

7. Wolf PA, Abbott RD, Kannel WB. "Atrial fibrillation as an independent risk factor for stroke: the Framingham Study." *Stroke*. 1991;22:983–988.

8. Camm AJ, Lip GY, De Caterina R, Savelieva I, Atar D, Hohnloser SH, et al.; ESC Committee for Practice Guidelines (CPG). "2012 focused update of the ESC Guidelines for the management of atrial fibrillation: an update of the 2010 ESC Guidelines for the management of atrial fibrillation. Developed with the special contribution of the European Heart Rhythm Association." *Eur Heart J*. 2012;33:2719–2747.

9- Eckman MH, Rosand J, Knudsen KA, Singer DE, Greenberg SM. "Can patients be anticoagulated after intracerebral hemorrhage? A decision analysis." *Stroke*. 2003;34:1710–1716.

10- Stoker TB, BChir MB, Evans NR. "Managing risk after intracerebral hemorrhage in concomitant atrial fibrillation and cerebral amyloid angiopathy." *Stroke*. 2016;47e190–e192.

23 Headache Following a New Medication

Bridget LaMonica Ostrem

Jane is a 19-year-old woman with a history of low-frequency episodic migraine who presents to clinic with a new headache type. She complains of daily holocephalic headaches for the past two weeks, with pain that is maximal upon awakening every morning. She also complains of photophobia and new episodes of brief visual darkening, "like a blanket covering my vision," which have increased in frequency and now occur up to fifteen times per day. Her typical migraine medications have not provided relief.

Medications are as-needed sumatriptan and ibuprofen, and daily minocycline, which was started two months ago for acne. On exam, vital signs are normal, BMI is 30.5 kg/m^2, and fundoscopy demonstrates bilateral papilledema. Her neurologic exam is otherwise normal.

What do I do now?

Diagnosis

A new type of headache in a patient with chronic migraine should prompt an evaluation for secondary etiologies. The finding of papilledema is concerning for increased intracranial pressure (ICP). Idiopathic intracranial hypertension (IIH) is a neurological disorder defined by increased ICP without an identifiable cause. Up to 80% of patients with IIH have headache. Additional symptoms include positive and negative visual phenomena, diplopia, tinnitus, and retroorbital pain. IIH occurs more frequently in women than men, with the highest incidence in women age 18–44 with obesity (up to 20 per 100,000). Other risk factors include recent weight gain, a family history of IIH, and medications such as tetracyclines, retinoids, and growth hormone. Several other conditions have known associations with IIH, although it has been suggested that these conditions increase the risk of obesity or occur in women with IIH risk factors without directly causing increased ICP. These conditions include polycystic ovarian syndrome, systemic lupus erythematosus, obstructive sleep apnea, and pregnancy. Jane has two risk factors: obesity and recent initiation of a tetracycline (minocycline).

Work-up

1. Neurological and neuro-ophthalmological examinations: When a patient presents with new headaches and papilledema, the first step in evaluation is a thorough exam to assess for other focal neurological deficits. The neurological exam is typically normal in IIH, although a cranial nerve VI palsy can occur with increased intracranial pressure. A neuro-ophthalmological exam is helpful in quantifying and following visual field deficits.
2. Neuroimaging (MRI and MR venogram) is required to rule out other causes of increased ICP. The differential includes a mass lesion, obstructive hydrocephalus, and venous sinus thrombosis. While imaging may be normal, findings associated with IIH include buckling of the optic nerve, optic nerve head protrusion and/or enhancement, flattening of the posterior aspect of the sclera, a partially empty sella, and transverse sinus stenosis (see Figure 23.1).

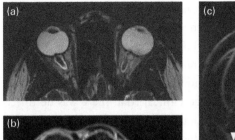
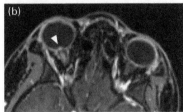
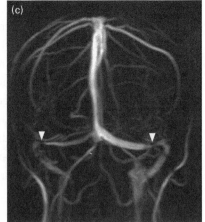

FIGURE 23.1 (A) MRI findings associated with IIH include protrusion of the optic nerve head and flattening of the posterior aspect of the sclera. (B) Enhancement of the optic nerve head. (C) Transverse sinus stenosis.

3. The next step in work-up is to obtain a lumbar puncture. Opening pressure should be measured in the lateral recumbent position, and a finding of >25 cm H_2O is considered elevated. Removal of 30cc–40cc of cerebrospinal fluid (CSF) often leads to rapid improvement in headache. Routine studies, including CSF glucose, protein, cell count, and gram stain and culture, are normal in patients with IIH. Abnormal findings should lead the clinician to search for an alternative diagnosis, such as lyme meningitis, which can present similarly to IIH with headache and elevated ICP.
4. Comorbidities such as anemia and obstructive sleep apnea should be evaluated and addressed.

IIH Treatment

Potentially contributing medications should be discontinued. In Jane's case, minocycline is stopped immediately.

While the initial lumbar puncture is usually therapeutic for patients with IIH, headache often returns within 24 hours, and persistently elevated ICP can lead to permanent vision loss. Repeat lumbar punctures may be needed.

If vision is rapidly worsening, surgical options should be considered such as lumbar drain, optic nerve sheath fenestration, or a shunt.

Most patients are started on a carbonic anhydrase inhibitor to reduce CSF production; common choices are topiramate and acetazolamide. In rats, topiramate was found to be more effective at reducing ICP than acetazolamide. In a small randomized clinical trial, there was no difference in term of improvement of visual field loss between topiramate up to 150 mg daily and acetazolamide doses up to 1500 mg daily.

Weight loss can also improve long-term visual outcomes. It can be very helpful to refer patients to a bariatric surgery/weight-loss management clinic.

Treatment of the Headache Attributed to IIH

There are no published randomized trials addressing the treatment of headache in IIH. However, topiramate is often used first, since it has proven efficacy in migraine and IIH and may help with IIH-related headache. Other migraine medications, including injections of botulinum toxin A, may be considered. Medications that can lead to weight gain and recurrent IIH should be avoided. It is also important to educate patients about the appropriate use of analgesic medications to prevent worsening of symptoms due to medication overuse headache.

Prognosis

While this condition was previously called benign intracranial hypertension, the name was changed to reflect the risk of significant morbidity in the form of disabling chronic pain and permanent vision loss. Patients with IIH commonly complain of persistent headache and visual symptoms for months to years. Improvement may be gradual and not complete. Symptoms may recur with additional weight gain, and permanent vision loss may occur. The headache may persist despite normalization of the ICP.

SPECIAL CONSIDERATIONS

Pregnancy

IIH can occur in pregnancy, but pregnancy is not a risk factor for IIH. When it happens, IIH most commonly occurs within the first half of pregnancy, though it can present during any trimester. There is an estimated prevalence in pregnant women of between 2% to 12%. Work-up follows the same progression as in nonpregnant patients, with MRI and MRV (without contrast) followed by lumbar puncture, which is safe to perform in pregnancy. Management includes repeat lumbar punctures and moderate weight reduction. If clinically indicated for IIH as a third line after reasonable weight control and serial lumbar punctures, acetazolamide can be considered with a risk-benefit discussion. Although it has been found to be associated with teratogenicity in animal studies where the dose used was much higher than in humans, there has not been documented human fetal risks to date. Acetazolamide and furosemide both used to be category C in pregnancy. Furosemide is associated with decreased placental perfusion, though, and should be avoided in pregnancy. Topiramate should be avoided in pregnancy due to teratogenicity such as increased risk of cleft palate. Topiramate used to be category D in pregnancy.

Several studies have found no evidence of increased abortion rate or altered perinatal outcomes among pregnant women with IIH. Neuraxial anesthesia can be safely given during labor and delivery. Visual outcomes are similar in pregnant and nonpregnant patients, and there are no contraindications to future pregnancies. Rates of recurrence are not elevated above that of nonpregnant patients with IIH.

Children

Infants as young as 4 months old have been reported with IIH. Obesity and female sex are demonstrated risk factors in postpubertal children; however, IIH occurs at approximately a 1:1 ratio in prepubertal boys and girls. Pediatric patients are less likely to complain of headache, and may present with vague, nonspecific symptoms such as nausea and vomiting. When performing lumbar puncture for opening pressure, a cutoff of 28 cm H_2O is considered elevated in children. Management is similar to adults, although weight loss or prevention of weight gain is only indicated in children with obesity.

KEY POINTS TO REMEMBER

- Idiopathic intracranial hypertension occurs most commonly in young women with obesity.
- Key steps in work-up are brain MRI and MR venogram followed by lumbar puncture measuring the opening pressure.
- Early recognition and management are key to decrease the risk of vision loss.
- Acute treatments, starting with lumbar puncture and occasionally including surgical management, are focused on rapid lowering of intracranial pressure.
- Long-term visual outcomes can be optimized with weight reduction and carbonic anhydrase inhibitors.

Further Reading

1. Mollan SP, Davies B, Silver NC, et al. "Idiopathic intracranial hypertension: consensus guidelines on management." *J Neurol Neurosurg Psychiatry*. 2018;89:1088–1100.
2. Wakerley BR, Tan MH, Ting EY. "Idiopathic intracranial hypertension." *Cephalalgia*. 2015;35(3):248–261. https://doi.org/10.1177/0333102414534329
3. Hingwala DR, Kesavadas C, Thomas B, Kapilamoorthy TR, Sarma PS. "Imaging signs in idiopathic intracranial hypertension: Are these signs seen in secondary intracranial hypertension too?" *Ann Indian Acad Neurol*. 2013;16(2):229–233. https://doi.org/10.4103/0972-2327.112476
4. NORDIC Idiopathic Intracranial Hypertension Study Group Writing Committee, Wall M, McDermott MP, Kieburtz KD, Corbett JJ, Feldon SE, Friedman DI, Katz DM, Keltner JL, Schron EB, Kupersmith MJ. "Effect of acetazolamide on visual function in patients with idiopathic intracranial hypertension and mild visual loss." *JAMA*. 2014;311(16):1641–1651. https://doi.org/10.1001/jama.2014.3312
5. Koc F, Isik MR, Sefi-Yurdakul N. "Weight reduction for a better visual outcome in idiopathic intracranial hypertension." *Arq Bras Oftalmol*. 2018;81(1):18–23. doi:10.5935/0004-2749.20180006
6. Aguiar M, et al. "The health economic evaluation of bariatric surgery versus a community weight management intervention analysis from the Idiopathic

Intracranial Hypertension Weight Trial (IIH:WT)." *Life* (Basel). vol. 2021;11(5):409. https://doi.org/10.3390/life11050409

7. Kesler A, Kupferminc M. "Idiopathic intracranial hypertension and pregnancy." *Clin Obstet Gynecol*. 2013;56(2):389–396. https://doi.org/10.1097/GRF.0b013e318 28f2701

8. Gaier ED, Heidary G. "Pediatric idiopathic intracranial hypertension." *Semin Neurol*. 2019;39(06):704–710. https://doi.org/10.1055/s-0039-1698743

24 In Search of a Durable Dural Patch

Elena Haight and Ian Carroll

A 19-year-old female with a history of lower extremity complex regional pain syndrome, but no signs of a hereditary disorder of connective tissue, presents complaining of daily occipital headaches that are better each morning, worsen with activity and as the day progresses; neck, shoulder, and interscapular pain; tachycardia with a resting heart rate in the 120s; and refractory nausea and vomiting. Notably, she had a spinal cord stimulator placed 3 years prior to presentation, which was complicated by unintended dural puncture with the 12-gauge introducer needle. She had no history of headache prior to her unintended dural puncture but developed an acute post–dural puncture headache (PDPH) that was felt to resolve with an epidural blood patch. However, months later, in the absence of any trauma or precipitating event, she experienced the gradual progressive onset of her current headache symptoms.

What do I do now?

Epidemiology

The absence of headaches prior to her previous dural punctures raises the suspicion of a chronic CSF leak, despite the fact that her headache is not obviously orthostatic, and she had been treated with an epidural blood patch (EBP) with apparent resolution of her acute PDPH.

CSF leak unrelated to PDPH is not rare—the estimated incidence of 5 per 100,000 makes it about as likely as pancreatic cancer and half as common as a subarachnoid hemorrhage or suicide, conditions commonly seen in a regional medical center.

Risk factors for atraumatic CSF leak and resulting spontaneous intracranial hypotension (SIH) include hereditary disorders of connective tissue, such as Marfan or Ehlers-Danlos syndrome, which may result in reduced structural integrity of the dura. Even in patients who do not meet criteria for known syndromes associated with hereditary disorders of connective tissue, patients with SIH and spontaneous CSF leak are more likely to have signs of abnormal connective tissue such as unusually tall stature, pectus abnormalities, benign joint hypermobility, or aortic dilatation and heart valve abnormalities. However, the degree to which a genetic predisposition plays a role in the recovery or failure to recover from a known dural puncture remains unknown.

Current data suggests that two-thirds of patients with spontaneous atraumatic CSF leak cannot identify a precipitating trauma or event. Among the one-third of patients that can identify a precipitating factor, these are often seemingly unimpressive, including: (1) stretching, Pilates, or yoga; (2) Valsalva maneuver from straining to lift, pass stool, cough, or vomit; and (3) bending over to lift something.

In this case, there was no history of a hereditary disorder of connective tissue nor obvious signs of such, though she was significantly taller than average and reported being more flexible than her friends as a child. The only potential precipitating factor was her known accidental dural puncture. Case control studies as well as prospective studies suggest that up to one-third of patients who experience an unintended dural puncture during placement of a labor epidural to facilitate childbirth will go on to experience new or worsened chronic headache. Similarly, about one-third of patients who develop an acute PDPH following planned spinal anesthesia may go on to develop chronic headache. Epidural blood patching appears to reduce, but not eliminate, this risk. Thus, her history of a dural puncture with a large bore needle puts her at risk for a chronic CSF leak.

Diagnosis

Persistent CSF leaks typically present differently than the acute CSF leak, though both may be spontaneous or traumatic. Whereas acute CSF leak is marked by orthostatic headache, chronic leaks typically have a less prominent orthostatic component. More prolonged time flat may be needed for only partial relief, and in some cases more prolonged time upright is needed to manifest peak intensity of head pain and pressure. Furthermore, chronic CSF leaks may present as a second-half of the day headache, exertional headache, non-orthostatic chronic daily headache, thunderclap headache, or reverse orthostatic headache. Head pain is typically but not exclusively bilateral and described in terms of "pressure." Discomfort is most characteristically localized to the occiput with spread to other areas of the head, face, and neck as intensity increases. CSF leaks are commonly accompanied by hearing alterations, tinnitus, vertigo, nausea, cognitive symptoms, and fatigue. Given the overlap in when these symptoms begin following a significant trauma, a patient may be diagnosed with post-concussion syndrome or mild traumatic brain injury, if the symptoms are not obviously orthostatic and imaging is negative.

Thus, characterizing the orthostatic nature of symptoms is critical and can be facilitated with a prescribed trial of prolonged recumbency. To this end, we often recommend that patients suspected of CSF leak numerically rate symptoms of head pain, neck pain, nausea, tinnitus, brain fog, and fatigue. Patients then lay flat for 24 or 48 hours prior to rating those same symptoms again while still flat. This allows quantification of the degree to which each symptom is orthostatic and allows circadian effects to be distinguished from postural effects that may be driving daily or late-day headaches.

Imaging can also facilitate diagnosis. Initial imaging should consist of a brain MRI and full spine with and without contrast. The mnemonic SEEPS has been used to describe classic signs of SIH on brain MRI: Subdural fluid collections, Enhancement of the pachymeninges, Engorgement of venous structures, Pituitary hyperemia, and Sagging of the brain (noted as cerebellar descent below the foramen magnum—potentially confused with

Chiari). More recently it has been appreciated that more subtle and perhaps markedly more sensitive signs include a reduced distance between the pituitary and the optic chiasm (suprasellar distance less than 4 mm); reduced distance from the pons to the clivus (prepontine distance less than 5 mm); and reduced distance from the mammillary body to the top of the pons (mammilopontine distance less the 6.5 mm). These should be measured on any brain MRI done to evaluate chronic refractory headache. Heavily weighted T2 MRI of the spine in the setting of CSF leak can reveal distention of the spinal epidural venous plexus, extradural fluid collections, abnormal intensity around nerve route sleeves, or even rents in the anterior dura from bone osteophytes and disc degeneration. Recent investigations suggest that 10%–25% of patients with orthostatic headache and totally normal brain and spine MRI can be demonstrated to have a CSF-venous fistula in which CSF leaks into an epidural vein. These findings highlight the limitations of MRI to exclude CSF leak. In this patient, MRI was precluded by her spinal cord stimulator, which was not MRI compatible.

Alternatives to MRI include radionuclide cisternography or CT myelogram. CT head is not generally useful in evaluating for CSF leak unless severe sagging is present. CT myelogram may be more useful than MRI for determining the source of a spinal fluid leak. CT myelography can also provide the opportunity to assess for CSF pressure and CSF protein. CSF protein is commonly elevated in patients with CSF leak, while CSF pressure may be low or normal. Research over the last decade suggests that as many as two-thirds of patients with imaging-proven CSF leaks have normal opening pressure, and 5% have opening pressure above 20 cc of water (i.e., elevated). Thus, a low opening pressure (less than 6 cm of water) should be viewed as specific but not sensitive—and used to rule in a leak. However, a normal opening pressure is not sensitive and cannot rule out a leak.

Treatment
In this case, a CT myelogram was initially unrevealing, and the patient was offered an empiric lumbar EBP. Data from patients with PDPH suggest higher volume 20cc–30cc patches are more successful than lower volume patches (15 cc or less), and this has been extrapolated to patients with spontaneous CSF leak. It is reasonable to try nondirected lumbar EBP as an initial approach, as localizing the site of the leak can be challenging even at

expert centers. When a nondirected EBP fails, localizing the leak becomes a priority to enable targeted EBP or targeted fibrin sealant epidural patches. Small retrospective case series suggest that as many as 50% of patients who fail to respond to EBP may respond to targeted fibrin sealant patches. Fibrin sealants expand after injection, and large volumes are avoided to reduce the risk of cord compression. We typically inject no more than 3 cc per level.

For this patient, EBP at the level of dural puncture from her spinal cord stimulator provided 3 weeks of relief from headache and nausea, and an associated decrease in resting HR from 120s to 80s, thus confirming the underlying diagnosis of CSF leak. The return of her symptoms after 3 weeks reflects a course consistent with chronic CSF leak, with 30% of patients responding to a single EBP and some 65%–75% responding to repeated EBP. Repeated EBP continued to provide the patient with relief that lasted only weeks to months. Though relatively safe, repeated EBP is not without risk, of which further dural tear, adhesive arachnoiditis, subdural or subarachnoid hematoma, seizures, and rebound intracranial hypertension are of greatest concern. A repeat CT myelogram revealed a dorsal dural bleb arising in aneurysmal fashion from the dorsal dura at the site of the spinal cord stimulator dural puncture. This was not visible on the previous CT myelogram due to the slightly different position of the relevant CT

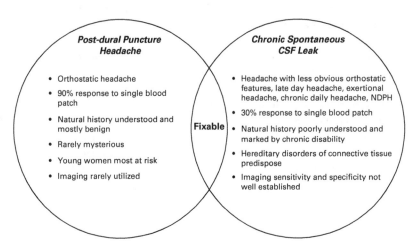

FIGURE 24.1 Key points to differentiate Post-dural Puncture Headache from Chronic Spontaneous CSF Leak.

acquisition slice. Visualization of this bleb allowed the patient to undergo successful open surgical repair, which confirmed this as the site of her leak.

KEY POINTS TO REMEMBER

- CSF leaks may occur spontaneously or after trauma.
- Chronic CSF leak may present as a second-half of the day headache, exertional headache, non-orthostatic chronic daily headache, thunderclap headache, or reverse orthostatic headache, and may be accompanied by neck pain, hearing alterations, tinnitus, vertigo, nausea, cognitive symptoms, and fatigue, whereas an acute CSF leak typically presents as orthostatic headache. (See Figure 24.1 for a useful diagnostic map.)
- Imaging studies such as brain MRI, spinal MRI, and CT and MR myelography can confirm the diagnosis of CSF leak but cannot definitively rule out a CSF leak.
- A single or repeated epidural blood patch is the standard of care for CSF leaks.

Further Reading

1. Häni L, Fung C, Jesse CM, et al. "Insights into the natural history of spontaneous intracranial hypotension from infusion testing." *Neurology.* 2020;95(3):e247–e255.
2. Schievink W. "Spontaneous intracranial hypotension." *New Engl J Med.* 2021;385:2173–2178.
3. Dobrocky T, Grunder L, Breiding P, et al. "Assessing Spinal cerebrospinal fluid leaks in spontaneous intracranial hypotension with a scoring system based on brain magnetic resonance imaging findings." *JAMA Neurol.* 2019;76(5):580–587.
4. D'Antona L, Jaime Merchan MA, Vassiliou A, et al. "Clinical presentation, investigation findings and treatment outcomes of spontaneous intracranial hypotension syndrome: a systematic review and meta-analysis." *JAMA Neurol.* 2021;78:329–337.

5. Mokri B, Hunter SF, Atkinson JLD, et al. "Orthostatic headaches caused by CSF leak but with normal CSF pressures." *Neurology*. 1998;51:786–790.

6. Kranz PG, Tanpitukpongse TP, Choudhury KR, et al. "How common is normal cerebrospinal fluid pressure in spontaneous intracranial hypotension?" *Cephalalgia*. 2016;36:1209–1217.

25 Is It All About Mass?

Kaitlyn Melnick, Ashley Parham Ghiaseddin, and Yulia Orlova

A 68-year-old woman with a remote history of migraine is in the emergency room with a headache that started a few weeks ago and has progressively worsened. Headache is diffuse, worse in the morning, and associated with nausea. Neurological exam was notable for subtle right dysmetria and optic disk swelling on fundoscopy. MRI brain revealed a 1cm right cerebellar brain tumor with significant peritumoral edema and early obstructive hydrocephalus.

She was treated with dexamethasone and had uneventful suboccipital craniotomy for tumor resection. At the time of routine follow-up 4 weeks later, she is complaining of a dull pressure around the incision. Her physical exam is normal, and her wound is well healed. Imaging showed expected post-surgical changes without signs of tumor recurrence, hemorrhage, infection, or hydrocephalus.

What do I do now?

This case presents a commonly feared scenario. Most patients with headache do not have brain tumors, and chances that brain neoplasm will be found as the cause of headache is less than 0.1% in otherwise healthy individuals presenting to general practitioners. In the emergency room, headache from serious conditions, including brain neoplasm, is seen more often (2%–13%). New onset of headache in a patient with known systemic cancer or abnormal neurological exam is always a warning sign for secondary cause, such as potential metastatic disease or primary brain tumor, and requires further evaluation.

Headache is the most common presenting complaint in children and young adults with brain tumor and is seen in 48% to 71% of patients. Headache secondary to brain tumor is more common in those with a history of primary headache disorder, infratentorial location, large size of the tumor, and midline shift.

Headache from brain tumor as the only symptom is uncommon (2%–16%) and usually presents with other signs, making thorough neurological exam and fundoscopy of the utmost importance.

The SNOOP4 mnemonic can be helpful to remember the warning signs of secondary headache, including brain tumor. S refers to systemic symptoms such as infection, cancer, and immunocompromised state; N reflects abnormal neurological symptoms, most commonly with seizures, weakness or confusion in brain tumor; two Os stand for onset as sudden thunderclap headache or a new headache in an older individual; four Ps reflect change in pattern, precipitated by Valsalva or postural changes, or presence of papilledema.

Contrary to historic belief, headache from brain neoplasm does not have specific characteristics. It can be intermittent, have tension type or migraine-like features. On rare occasions, trigeminal autonomic cephalalgia can be associated with secreting pituitary tumors and neoplasms involving cavernous sinus or posterior fossa. Location of pain usually does not reflect location of tumor, except when headache is strictly unilateral and side locked, which can indicate the presence of ipsilateral brain tumor.

There are multiple mechanisms of headache in patients with neoplasm. The main mechanisms are local and distal traction of dura and pain-sensitive intracranial vessels; direct compression of intracranial portions of trigeminal, glossopharyngeal, vagus and upper cervical nerves C1, C2, or C3; mass effect; and hydrocephalus. Peripheral sensitization from neurogenic inflammation and central sensitization through trigeminovascular afferents can also contribute to prolonged headache, which can provide a link to shared pathophysiology between primary and secondary headache disorders.

Our patient had history of migraine in the past, but the recent onset of progressive headache was different. She also had focal findings on exam and optic disc swelling, which raised suspicion for space-occupying lesion.

Once red flags for secondary headache are identified and a brain tumor is suspected, brain magnetic resonance imaging (MRI) with and without contrast should be performed. MRI is superior to computed tomography (CT) in neoplasm detection, especially in the posterior fossa location. Following the discovery of a new brain mass, the patient should have complete workup for malignancy. The patient should be referred to a neurosurgeon for evaluation and may also need to be seen by an oncologist and radiation oncologist. If metastatic disease is suspected, identification of a primary tumor and systemic disease burden is important. Large tumors with significant mass effect (typically greater than 1 cm) and impending herniation should be expedited via admission to the hospital.

Treatment of headache secondary to neoplasm depends on tumor type, disease stage, and functional status of the patient. Surgical resection of tumor, radiotherapy, and/or chemotherapy may improve headache. Whole brain radiation can provide symptomatic relief for patients with metastatic disease in some cases.

Our patient had significant peritumoral edema, so corticosteroids were started as a temporary measure to reduce vasogenic edema. Dexamethasone is most used, and dose should be titrated to clinical effect, which is not immediate and becomes apparent in 24 to 72 hours. Common side effects include hyperglycemia, insomnia, and agitation. Peptic ulceration can be prevented by using proton pump inhibitors or histamine 2 receptor blockers. Chronic steroid treatment can also cause steroid-induced myopathy and infection. Steroids are typically weaned postoperatively over 1–2 weeks.

For moderate to severe pain, opioids and butalbital-containing medications can provide temporary relief, but prolonged use of these medications is associated with additional health risks, including dependence, respiratory depression, and medication overuse headache, especially in patients with coexistent primary headache disorders. Migraine-like headache can be treated with triptans, if not contraindicated. Simple analgesics and nonsteroidal anti-inflammatory (NSAIDs) medications can be used for symptomatic relief of mild headache. NSAIDs are contraindicated in patients with renal failure and peptic ulcer disease and are generally avoided before surgical treatment due to potential increased risk of bleeding. Because of hepatotoxicity risk, dose of acetaminophen should not exceed 4 to 6 grams daily. Triptans can be helpful in those with migraine-like headache, but they should not be overused.

When headache persists or develops after craniotomy, several etiologies should be considered. Cervicogenic headache due to positioning during surgery; headache from cerebrospinal fluid leak; infections such as meningitis, cerebritis, or ventriculitis; hydrocephalus; and intracranial hemorrhage can develop in the immediate postoperative period. When headache persists, tumor recurrence or radiation necrosis can be potential causes. Patients who had radiation therapy may develop a syndrome of stroke-like migraine attacks after radiation therapy (SMART) years later, with attacks of prolonged neurological deficit and migraine-like headache. Delayed effect of brain radiation can also present as peri-ictal pseudo-progression (PIPG) and acute late-onset encephalopathy after radiation therapy (ALERT) syndrome. In many of these scenarios, repeat imaging is prudent. Chemotherapy drugs (temozolamide, bevacizumab), antiemetics (ondansetron), and withdrawal from steroids can also cause headache.

Up to 60% of patients have post-craniotomy headache (PCH), which is more frequent after suboccipital surgery. Multiple mechanisms of PCH are proposed that include not only local factors such as surgical trauma, cranial nerves injury, or development of neurinomas in the surgical scar, but also central sensitization. Various preoperative strategies that include scalp nerve blocks, gabapentinoids, and steroids are employed to reduce acute post-craniotomy. Most commonly it is short lived and completely resolves, but some patients develop persistent PCH that lasts longer than 3 months, in which case preventive therapy targeting clinical phenotype should be considered, although there is insufficient data on the utility of this strategy.

Patients with lancinating post-craniotomy pain may have relief from carbamazepine or oxcarbazepine. For neuropathic pain, gabapentinoids (gabapentin, pregabalin), anticonvulsants (lamotrigine, topiramate, tiagabine), and tricyclic antidepressants (amitriptyline, nortriptyline) can be helpful.

In a patient with clinical phenotype consistent with migraine, preventive therapy with anticonvulsants (valproate, topiramate), antihypertensives (beta-blockers), and antidepressants (amitriptyline, venlafaxine) can be tried. Treatment of underlying primary headache disorder with standard therapy should not be overlooked.

Anticonvulsants valproate and topiramate can have additional benefit for mood stabilization and seizures prophylaxis, but they are also associated with side effects. Hepatotoxicity and weight gain, especially when used with steroids, are side effects of valproate that should be monitored. Topiramate can cause weight loss, which can limit its use when patients have poor appetite related to cytotoxic chemotherapy. Gabapentinoids overall are well tolerated, but at high doses can cause sedation. Beta-blockers such as atenolol, metoprolol, and propranolol should be avoided in patients with poorly controlled asthma and COPD, because they can worsen respiratory function.

The patient in our case can benefit from initiation of gabapentin for her headache because of the neuropathic features of her headache. If her headache persists and she develops migraine-like features, the headache may respond to medications used for migraine prophylaxis.

KEY POINTS TO REMEMBER

- Most patients with headache do not have brain tumor, but many patients with brain tumor have headache.
- Evaluation of patients with headache should start with screening for red flags for secondary headache.
- Headache from brain tumor is rarely an isolated symptom, and there are usually diagnostic clues on clinical history, neurological exam, and fundoscopy.
- Most headaches from brain tumor resolve after treatment of tumor.
- When headache persists, preventive treatment according to headache phenotype should be offered.

Disclosures:

Dr. Ghiaseddin has received personal fees from Monteris Medical and Novocure; research funding support from Orbus Therapeutics.

Further Reading

1. Forsyth PA, Posner JB. Intracranial neoplasms. In: Olesen J, Tfelt-Hansen P, Welch KMA, editors. *The Headaches*. 2nd edition. New York: Raven Press; 2000. pp. 849–859.
2. Loghin M, Levin VA. "Headache related to brain tumors." *Curr Treat Options Neurol*. 2006;8:21–32.
3. Dodick DW. "Pearls: headache." *Semin Neurol*. 2010;30:74–81.
4. Taylor LP. "Mechanism of brain tumor headache." *Headache*. 2014;54:772–775.
5. Lutman B, Bloom J, Nussenblatt B, Romo V. "A contemporary perspective on the management of post-craniotomy headache and pain." *Curr Pain Headache Rep*. 2018;22: 69.
6. Kirby S, Purdy RA. "Headaches and brain tumors." *Neurol Clin*. 2014;32:423–432.

26 Unexpected Findings in the Sella

Eric A. Kaiser

A 32-year-old woman with no significant past
medical history presents to your clinic complaining
of worsening headaches. She reports developing
headaches associated with photophobia and nausea
as a teenager. Prior headaches typically occurred
a few times a month and terminated with over-
the-counter analgesics. However, over the past
several months she states her headaches have
become daily and no longer respond to simple
analgesics. Headaches are currently described as
left-sided periorbital and frontal, throbbing pain with
associated photophobia, phonophobia, and nausea.
On examination, patient has full visual fields by
confrontation, intact cranial nerves, and otherwise
normal neurologic examination. You recommend that
she obtain a brain MRI due to the progressive nature
of her headaches. A few weeks later the MRI report
describes a 6 mm pituitary lesion consistent with a
pituitary microadenoma.

What do I do now?

Incidental Pituitary Neuroendocrine Tumors (Adenomas)

One could argue that your patient presented with worsening headache; thus this pituitary incidentaloma by definition is not incidental, as the MRI was prompted by headache, which may or may not be secondary to the lesion. Nevertheless, incidental pituitary lesions are found in 0.1% to 1.2% of MRI brain examinations and detected in 10% of MRI pituitary examinations. Postmortem studies have estimated 11% to 23% of the population have pituitary lesions. The most common lesions are Rathke's cleft cysts (which rarely grow) and pituitary neuroendocrine tumors, more commonly referred to as adenomas; but rare lesions are possible, including pituitary metastases, hemorrhages, infarctions, epidermoid cysts, and abscesses. Craniopharyngiomas and meningiomas may invade the sella and appear to be part of the hypophysis. Pituitary glands that are heterogenous on imaging may also mimic a pituitary lesion.

Pituitary adenomas have been arbitrarily classified as macroadenomas for lesions >10 mm in size or microadenomas (incidentalomas) for lesions <10 mm in size. Macroadenomas are rarely found incidentally, as they are typically symptomatic, often causing hypopituitarism or neurologic complications from compression of the optic chiasm or nerves, leading to visual field loss or invasion of the cavernous sinus, or optic apex leading to ophthalmoplegia.

Work-up

After reviewing the MRI findings, you follow up with the patient to discuss the results and ask about signs and symptoms suggestive of hormone hypersecretion (Table 26.1) and hypopituitarism. Although the patient denies any signs or symptoms, you recommend a comprehensive lab work-up (as outlined in Table 26.1) to determine whether the microadenoma is oversecreting. One-third of pituitary adenomas are clinically nonfunctioning. For those that are oversecreting tumors, half are prolactinomas, and the remainder are growth hormone- or ACTH-secreting tumors. Less than 1% of pituitary adenomas are thyrotropin-secreting adenomas. If the tumor is 6 mm or larger, then you should evaluate for hypopituitarism (including free T4, morning cortisol, and testosterone levels; other tests to consider include TSH, LH, FSH, and IGF-1). Lab work for this patient is unremarkable. However, if there is evidence of an oversecreting adenoma or

TABLE 26.1 Clinical symptoms of oversecreting pituitary adenomas and hormone levels to check for each type.

	Symptoms	Hormones Levels to Check
Prolactinoma (Prolactin-secreting Tumor)	loss of libido, erectile dysfunction, infertility oligomenorrhea or amenorrhea, galactorrhea, osteoporosis	Prolactin levels
Acromegaly (Growth Hormone-secreting Tumor)	diabetes mellitus, hypertension, sleep apnea, arthritis, carpal tunnel syndrome, facial features changes (prognathism, enlargement of lip, tongue, & nose), gigantism (if onset prior to closure of epiphyses during puberty)	Growth hormone IGF-1 level
Cushing Disease (ACTH-Secreting Tumor)	hypercortisolism—weight gain, redistribution of fat (centripetal obesity, increases supra- and dorsocervical fat pads), facial rounding, violaceous skin striae and ecchymoses, diabetes mellitus, hypertension, depression and other mood disorders, osteoporosis	Late-night salivary cortisol level Overnight 1 mg dexamethasone suppression test 24-hr urinary free cortisol
Thyrotropin-secreting Tumor	hyperthyroidism—weight loss, tachycardia and arrhythmias, sweating, increase appetite, irritability, anxiety, goiter	Thyroxine level (T4) Triiodothyronine (T3) levels Thyrotropin (thyroid-stimulating hormone, TSH) level
Clinically nonfunctioning adenomas	asymptomatic or symptoms secondary to mass effect including headaches, visual field deficits, ophthalmoplegias, hypopituitarism	

hypopituitarism, referral to endocrinology is appropriate for further evaluation and management. For prolactinomas, medical therapy with dopamine agonists (e.g., cabergoline) is used initially for treatment, as they may decrease tumor size. If the tumor abuts the optic chiasm, then refer for visual field–testing. If no deficits, continue monitor visual fields closely every 6 to 12 months.

Monitoring

Currently, it appears that your patient's microadenoma is clinically non-functioning and asymptomatic. You recommend monitoring with repeat MRI imaging in 12 months. For lesions >10 mm, repeat imaging should be performed at 6 months. MR imaging should include thin-cuts through the pituitary gland, with and without contrast. Imaging should be repeated every 12 months for the next 3 years, and gradually less frequently thereafter to monitor for tumor growth. Only 10% of incidental microadenomas will grow, and there have been no cases of microadenomas enlarging to the point of compression or invasion. In addition to imaging, lab work-up for hypopituitarism should be repeated in 6 months and then every 12 months thereafter for macroadenomas, or when there is evidence of tumor enlargement or changes in clinical course.

Indications for Neurosurgery Referral

For those tumors that show significant pituitary enlargement to 10 mm or larger in size, or evidence of GH, ACHT or TSH oversecretion, refer to an expert pituitary neurosurgeon for consideration of transsphenoidal resection. Also consider neurosurgical referral if there is evidence of hypopituitarism, visual field deficits, ophthalmoplegia, or other neurologic deficits secondary to tumor invasion or compression. For patients who are not surgical candidates, radiotherapy and medical therapy may be considered. Hemorrhage into pituitary adenomas (i.e., pituitary apoplexy) only occurs in macroadenomas and is a rare complication (7.3%–9.5% of cases), but anticoagulation may increase this risk.

In a follow-up visit, the patient asks whether her headaches are due to her pituitary adenoma and whether her headaches would resolve with surgery. Teasing out whether her headache is secondary to the lesion or a primary headache can be tricky. In a 2015 study by Rizzoli and colleagues, 63%

(n = 84) of patients referred to a multidisciplinary neuroendocrine clinic for suspected pituitary lesions reported recurrent headaches. Participants reporting headaches were more likely to be female and have a prior headache diagnosis. Headaches were most commonly described as unilateral (71%) with an anterior localization (frontal, temporal, or retro-orbital; 82%) and were often associated with migrainous features or less often with features of trigeminal autonomic cephalalgias. After surgical resection, headache resolved in 35% (9/26) and improved in 46% (12/26) of patients who reported recurrent headache preoperatively. Careful assessment of a preexisting primary headache disorder may aid in determining whether the headache is secondary to the pituitary lesion. While unremitting headache has been suggested as a potential indication for surgical resection, optimizing medical management of the headache first may avoid resection if headache is the only indication for surgery.

KEY POINTS TO REMEMBER

- Pituitary neuroendocrine tumors (adenomas) are common incidental findings on MRI brain.
- Work-up for pituitary adenomas, regardless of size, should include hormone levels to determine if the tumor is oversecreting or causing hypopituitarism.
- Refer to endocrinology if the tumor is prolactin-secreting or additional medical work-up or management is needed.
- For tumors that abut the optic chiasm or nerves, obtain visual field testing.
- Refer to a pituitary neurosurgeon for transsphenoidal resection if the tumor is >10 mm or oversecreting GH, ACHT, or TSH, or if there is evidence of hypopituitarism, visual field deficit, or ophthalmoplegia.
- If monitoring for tumor growth, MR imaging should be repeated at 6 months for tumors >10 mm or 12 months for tumors <10 mm, and repeated annually for at least 3 years.

Further Reading

1. Freda PU, Beckers AM, Katznelson L, et al. "Pituitary incidentaloma: an endocrine society clinical practice guideline." *J Clin Endocrinol Metab.* 2011;96(4):894–904.
2. Molitch ME. "Diagnosis and treatment of pituitary adenomas: a review." *JAMA.* 2017;317(5):516–524.
3. Hoang JK, Hoffman AR, Gonzalez RG, et al. "Management of incidental pituitary findings on CT, MRI, and (18)f-fluorodeoxyglucose PET: a white paper of the ACR Incidental Findings Committee." *J Am Coll Radiol.* 2018;15(7):966–972.
4. Rizzoli P, Iuliano S, Weizenbaum E, Laws E. "Headache in patients with pituitary lesions: a longitudinal cohort study." *Neurosurgery.* 2016;78(3):316–323.

27 Day-in, Day-out

Olivia Begasse de Dhaem and Carolyn Bernstein

A 40-year-old mother of three young children with no past medical history wants to establish care to renew her fioricet refills. Her mother and sister also have headaches, but no diagnosis. Her headaches started after the birth of her first child and improved during her subsequent pregnancies, but recurred postpartum. She prioritizes her family over self-care and seldom goes to the doctor. She self-medicated with three cups of coffee daily and ibuprofen almost every day for years, until she once went to the emergency room for a headache that was more severe than her prior headaches in terms of pain intensity. Basic blood work and head CT without contrast were unremarkable. She was given IV fluids, metoclopramide, magnesium, and dexamethasone, and was discharged on fioricet as needed. Since fioricet was so helpful in treating her headaches, she asked her primary care doctor for more prescriptions. She has now taken at least 3 fioricets per day for the last 2 years. Her doctor retired, so now she needs someone else to send prescriptions for her.

What do I do now?

Diagnosis

She does not have any red flags, so there is no need for further work-up. Her initial headaches met criteria for migraine (lasting the whole day until she slept them off in a quiet dark room, moderate to severe throbbing pain leading to avoidance of any physical activity, associated with photophobia and phonophobia). Since she grew up around family members who had similar headaches, she thought that her headaches were "normal" and did not know she had migraine.

She does meet ICHD-3 criteria for medication overuse headache (MOH) due to both fioricet and ibuprofen. She has a preexisting headache disorder (migraine); has a headache at least 15 days per month; and has been frequently taking acute medications for more than 3 months, which has been associated with an aggravation in her headaches. Most people with MOH have a prior history of migraine or tension-type headache. The MOH phenotype depends on the preexisting headache. Although combination analgesics are thought to be the most common culprits, different classes of acute treatments are involved in MOH. The frequency of acute medication intake to meet ICHD-3 criteria for MOH varies based on the medication class. Intake of at least 10 days per month is required for ergotamine, triptan, opioid, combination analgesic, multiple drug classes not individually overused. Intake of at least 15 days per month is required for acetaminophen, NSAIDs, and other non-opioid analgesics. However, there is not the best quality of evidence to justify those cut-offs and there may be individual variations in their susceptibility to MOH. Of note, rimegepant is the first medication used for both acute and preventive treatment of migraine. As such, rimegepant is thought to not be associated with MOH. Since she meets ICHD-3 criteria for both chronic migraine and MOH, she should be given both diagnoses.

Education

The concept of medication overuse headache is controversial because (1) it places an unfair and unfounded blame on patients, (2) it comes with the pitfall of unjustified undertreatment to "avoid" MOH, which leads to even more suffering, and (3) there is not strong evidence to support a causal effect of medication "overuse" and headaches. Sadly, some patients are reluctant to treat their migraine attacks early and aggressively out of fear of developing MOH. They should really take acute treatment as needed and as early as possible without guilt, while their providers help optimize their preventive therapies and provide support and reassurance. Dr. Young and his colleagues are recommending the term *medication adaptation headache* (MAH) to focus on the mechanism of the headache and avoid unjustified blame. If using the term MOH, it is essential to explain patients it is NOT their fault, explain the principles of acute and preventive therapy, and offer options to optimize treatment. Although not completely understood, the theoretical mechanism for MAH is long-term frequent acute treatment leading to suppression of endogenous antinociceptive systems, and hence upregulation of the calcitonin gene-related peptide (CGRP) system, which then facilitates the trigeminal nociceptive process. It is important to offer preventive medications to patients as soon as they are clinically eligible, to try to avoid the need for frequent acute medication use in the first place.

Management

To date, there is no formal consensus on optimal management. The management generally consists of (1) starting a preventive treatment and discussing behavioral techniques such as sleep hygiene and regular exercise, and (2) keeping track of headache days and medication use in a calendar or application. Reducing the frequency and severity of attacks will help decrease acute treatment use and will help with the anxiety of future attacks, and hence the mental need to stay ahead of the curve. Evaluating for and addressing potential comorbidities such as depression may also help.

Opiate or butalbital–containing agents should be tapered off. They are not recommended acute treatments for migraine nor tension-type headaches. They are associated with impaired alertness, dependence, and addiction. Be cautious of fioricet withdrawal, which may lead to seizures. For people who take 3 fioricets daily, progressively tapering off the fioricet may be enough. However, for people who take more fioricets daily, weaning off with a phenobarbital taper is safer, as it has a longer half-life. The conversion is 30 mg of phenobarbital for 100 mg butalbital (2 fioricets). The conversion is for seizure prevention; it will not help with the headaches. The doses of phenobarbital are slowly decreased every day.

Abrupt withdrawal of other potentially offending medications is recommended. When stopping an acute medication, the severity of MAH attacks may initially worsen. Bridge therapy with triptans, NSAIDs with longer half-lives such as nabumetone, DHE, steroids, or depakote can help during that time. Ultimately, detoxification may lead to a decreased headache frequency and improved acute and preventive treatment efficacy, especially if combined with preventive therapy. Not everyone will get better after the "washout period," which then questions the initial MAH diagnosis. Detoxification may not be needed for patients started on CGRP monoclonal antibodies, topiramate, or onabotulinum toxin A. There is no consensus on the timing of detoxification and prevention. Complete detoxification is not necessarily needed, as long as PRN use is limited to less than 2 days per week.

We cannot stress enough the importance of thoroughly explaining and discussing the plan with patients. The plan to address MAH needs to have strategies and enough medications for patients to treat their headaches as needed. The goal is not to increase suffering. Bridge therapy should be offered when the plan is expected to bring a worsening of headaches at first.

KEY POINTS TO REMEMBER

- MAH only occurs in people with a preexisting headache disorder.
- Optimize headache management. Remove any sense of blame from the patient.
- Progressively taper off opiate and barbiturate-containing agents.
- Start pharmacological and non-pharmacological preventive therapies.
- Evaluate and address potential comorbidities.
- Educate patients on MAH, our current understanding of its mechanism, treatment plan, and expectations.

Further Reading

1. Solomon M, Nahas SJ, Segal JZ, Young WB. "Medication adaptation headache." *Cephalalgia.* 2011;31(5):515–517. https://doi.org/10.1177/0333102410387678

2. Scher AI, Rizzoli PB, Loder EW. "Medication overuse headache: an entrenched idea in need of scrutiny." *Neurology*. 2017;89(12):1296–1304. https://doi.org/10.1212/WNL.0000000000004371

3. Diener HC, Holle D, Solbach K, Gaul C. "Medication-overuse headache: risk factors, pathophysiology and management." *Nat Rev Neurol*. 2016;12(10):575–583. https://doi.org/10.1038/nrneurol.2016.124

4. Carlsen LN, Munksgaard SB, Nielsen M, et al. "Comparison of 3 treatment strategies for medication overuse headache: a randomized clinical trial." *JAMA Neurol*. 2020;77(9):1069–1078. https://doi.org/10.1001/jamaneurol.2020.1179

5. Sun-Edelstein C, et al. "The evolution of medication overuse headache: history, pathophysiology and clinical update." *CNS Drugs*. 2021;35(5):545–565. https://doi.org/10.1007/s40263-021-00818-9

6. Meskunas CA, et al. "Medications associated with probable medication overuse headache reported in a tertiary care headache center over a 15-year period." *Headache*. 2006;46(5):766–772. https://doi.org/10.1111/j.1526-4610.2006.00442.x

28 I'm Not Sick Anymore!: Why Am I Still Having Headaches?

Ashley Alex

Jane is a 34-year-old intensive care unit nurse with a history of multiple sclerosis who presents for headaches that have been ongoing for the past 6 months since having tested positive for severe acute respiratory syndrome coronavirus 2 (SARS-CoV-2). At the time of diagnosis, she also experienced fever, chills, generalized fatigue, diarrhea, and ageusia, but only the headaches have persisted. Headache episodes are characterized by sudden onset, severe shooting pain radiating from the bilateral occipital region up toward the top of her head, with superimposed frontal pressure. They are often accompanied by irritability, photophobia, and allodynia. Headache attacks have led to disability resulting in missed days of work. General and neurologic examinations are unremarkable, including normal fundoscopy. Her mother has a history of intracranial aneurysm, which is disconcerting to the patient.

What do I do now?

Diagnosis

The most important and initial step of headache diagnosis is to always rule out secondary etiologies. A detailed history and physical examination including fundoscopy is vital to look for red flags such as mental status changes, focal neurological deficits, and evidence of increased intracranial pressure. Given the new sudden-onset headache, especially with the history of aneurysm in a first-degree relative, aneurysmal bleed should be considered in the differential. Reversible infectious etiologies such as meningitis or encephalitis are on the differential, and a lumbar puncture with opening pressure and cerebrospinal fluid analysis should be considered if there are clinical signs. When such red flags are present, magnetic resonance imaging (MRI) of the brain with and without gadolinium should be obtained to evaluate for any structural abnormalities, evidence of infection, signs of increased intracranial pressure, and so on.

Jane is diagnosed with headache attributed to coronavirus disease 2019 (COVID-19) infection. The International Classification of Headache Disorders, 3rd edition (ICHD-3) defines headache attributed to systemic viral infection as headaches "caused by and occurring in association with other symptoms and/or clinical signs of a systemic viral infection," and other secondary causes must be ruled out first. The headache is expected to develop at the same time as the systemic viral infection, worsen with worsening of systemic viral infection, and improve with improvement/resolution of systemic viral infection. The headache should be diffuse and/or moderate/severe in intensity.

Pathophysiology

Headache is one of the most common symptoms of COVID-19 due to severe acute respiratory SARS-CoV-2. Multiple mechanisms have been proposed as potential causes of headache related to COVID-19 infection. These include direct invasion of the central nervous system or invasion through the glia, coagulopathy, inflammation secondary to cytokines and inflammatory mediators, increased calcitonin gene-related peptide (CGRP) release, hypoxemia, dehydration, and metabolic disturbances.

Characteristics

Headaches associated with COVID-19 may serve as an important prognostic indicator, as they correlate with lower mortality and 7-day shorter disease course. They may be seen at any stage and may be persistent even after the acute infection has resolved. Headaches tend to range in severity, with those reported as severe more often identified as a prodromal symptom and observed more frequently in women and younger patients. The pain is typically bilateral and is either generalized or located frontotemporally. Even in those with preexisting headache disorders, the severity, duration, and/or rapid onset differentiate it from others. The headaches were described as a pressing or pulsating sensation aggravated by activity and more resistant to common analgesics. Fever was found to be the most frequent trigger, and the headaches were more closely related to anosmia, ageusia, and gastrointestinal complaints.

Treatment

Treatment of the headache should be directed toward the underlying cause. If none is identified, then treatment should be aimed toward the phenotype of the headache. To date, there are no trials for the treatment of headache attributed to COVID-19 infection.

Acute treatments for the headache associated with COVID-19 infection include nonsteroidal anti-inflammatory drugs (NSAIDs), steroids, triptans if there is no evidence of stroke or other cardiovascular contraindication, gepants, anti-emetics, and even muscle relaxants. While there was initial concern regarding the use of NSAIDs given that they upregulate the expression of angiotensin-converting enzyme 2 (ACE2) and could theoretically increase the risk for infection, there has been no substantial evidence to support this.

For frequent and/or disabling headaches, preventive therapies should be considered to decrease the overall severity and frequency. For those with a migrainous phenotype, preventive treatments include amitriptyline, onabotulinumtoxinA (botox) and CGRP monoclonal antibodies. The CGRP monoclonal antibodies could target the increased circulating levels of CGRP that occur as a result of the unchecked action of angiotensin II. Devices may also be a non-pharmacologic option to treat head pain;

noninvasive vagus nerve stimulators may help downregulate the inflammatory cytokine storm associated with COVID-19.

KEY POINTS TO REMEMBER

- It is imperative to rule out secondary headache disorders with appropriate imaging and diagnostic tests.
- Presence of headaches associated with COVID-19 may indicate a more benign and shorter disease course.
- Headaches may vary but are most typically bilateral, frontotemporal, moderate to severe intensity, and resistant to simple analgesics.
- Headaches associated with COVID-19 tend to be more closely associated with fever, diarrhea, anosmia, and ageusia.
- Treatment should be targeted at the underlying phenotype of the headaches with a combination of preventive and acute therapies.

Further Reading

1. Bolay H, Gül A, Baykan B. "COVID-19 is a real headache!" *Headache*. 2020;60(7):1415–1421. https://doi.org/10.1111/head.13856
2. Caronna E, Ballvé A, Llauradó A, et al. "Headache: a striking prodromal and persistent symptom, predictive of COVID-19 clinical evolution." *Cephalalgia*. 2020;40(13):1410–1421. https://doi.org/10.1177/0333102420965157
3. Caronna E, Pozo-Rosich P. "Headache as a symptom of COVID-19: narrative review of 1-year research." *Curr Pain Headache Rep*. 2021;25(11):73. https://doi.org/10.1007/s11916-021-00987-8
4. Tolebeyan AS, Zhang N, Cooper V, Kuruvilla DE. "Headache in patients with severe acute respiratory syndrome coronavirus 2 infection: a narrative review." *Headache*. 2020;60(10):2131–2138. https://doi.org/10.1111/head.13980
5. Messlinger K, et al. "Activation of the trigeminal system as a likely target of SARS-CoV-2 may contribute to anosmia in COVID-19." *Cephalalgia*. 2022;42(2):176–180.

29 All My Stress Goes to My Neck

Mohammad Hadi Gharedaghi and Julie H. Huang-Lionnet

Jane is a 37-year-old woman with endometriosis, interstitial cystitis, temporal mandibular joint disorder, general anxiety disorder, panic disorder, post-traumatic stress disorder, and an extensive family history of substance abuse, who presents with right-sided, non-throbbing pain radiating from her right upper neck and occipital region, spreading anteriorly to the orbital and frontal regions. Although fluctuating in severity, her pain is continuous and of moderate intensity on average. It is associated with right-sided neck tension and limited range of motion on neck rotation, flexion, and extension. Her headache worsens on head turning and digital palpation of neck muscles on the right. She did have a car accident 10 years ago when she briefly lost consciousness. Non-contrast CTs of the head and cervical spine were unremarkable at the time. She started to notice the pain 9 months ago when she lost her job. She does not have any autoimmune, endocrine, or rheumatological disorder.

What do I do now?

Diagnosis

The first step is to rule out any secondary concerning causes such as an arterial dissection, posterior cranial fossa lesion, or meningitis. She does not have any red flags, paresthesia, sensory or motor changes, or deep tendon reflex abnormalities. The pain onset was not acute, and the pain intensity waxes and wanes. She is afebrile. She has no skin rash. There is no evidence of scoliosis, and palpation of the spinous processes is not painful.

Cervicogenic headache is a syndrome that can be caused by different underlying disorders of the bony, disc, or soft tissue parts of the upper cervical spine usually associated with neck pain, such as tumors, fractures, and rheumatoid arthritis. Cervical myofascial trigger points are not valid causes for cervicogenic headache according to the ICHD-3 diagnostic criteria. Headaches related to cervical myofascial trigger points are usually coded as tension-type headaches associated with pericranial tenderness, but the ICHD-3 appendix differential of headache attributed to cervical myofascial pain may also be used. Of note, ICHD-3 appendix diagnoses have to be either confirmed or refuted. Similarly, C2 or C3 radiculopathy is not a valid cause for cervicogenic headache; the diagnosis of headache attributed to upper cervical radiculopathy appears in the ICHD-3 appendix.

Cervicogenic headaches are typically described as dull, non-pulsating, pressure, tightness, and non-throbbing in character. Other headache conditions may share similar posterior distribution secondary to the convergent anatomic pathways of upper cervical (C1–C3) and trigeminal nociceptive afferents with varying descriptions of the headache quality.

Other considerations on the differential include side-locked primary headaches, but Jane does not meet the autonomic features, temporality, location, and restlessness of trigeminal autonomic cephalalgias. Migraine can present with neck tension and some features of cervicogenic headache, but to a lesser extent. She also does not have migrainous features such as photophobia, phonophobia, nausea, vomiting, or throbbing pain. Migrainous features, however, may be present with cervicogenic headaches although not as typical and to a lesser extent than seen in migraine. Jane does not meet the temporal criteria of a persistent headache attributed to traumatic injury to the head (the headache did not develop within 7 days of the accident).

MANAGEMENT

Jane was prescribed a short course of low-dose tizanidine and referred to neck physical therapy. Neck physical therapy is the first-line treatment approach to cervicogenic headache. She was also advised to apply heat to her painful neck areas and do the daily exercises recommended by her physical therapist. Manual therapy does not seem to add any additional benefit.

At follow-up a month later, she had minimal improvement. An MRI of the cervical spine was ordered to rule out structural secondary etiologies and evaluate the facet joints. The underlying etiology of cervicogenic headache has to be addressed. Pain from the C2–C3 zygapophysial joint is common after whiplash injury and can spread from the occipital region to the frontal region and orbit. Jane had a history of neck trauma, which is reported in about one-third of patients with cervicogenic headache and may contribute to facet joint injury.

Jane was referred to an interventional pain doctor. A fluoroscopically guided third occipital nerve block significantly reduced her pain, including the pain in the frontal and orbital areas, which had both diagnostic and treatment value. Below C2–C3, facet joints are supplied by the medial branch of the dorsal ramus above and below. Hence, fluoroscopically guided medial branch blocks are performed for diagnosis and treatment. Although physical examination is often reported as a means to identify a painful facet joint, clinical studies have now revealed that prognostic blocks are the best approach to selecting patients for treatment. To date, no pharmacological treatment has proven effective for the treatment of cervicogenic headache, including onabotulinum toxin A injections into neck muscles. Radiofrequency denervation is the standard treatment for facet joint pain, with moderate evidence supporting its efficacy.

Comorbidities including mood and chronic pain disorders should be addressed, as they contribute to pain sensitization and chronification. Jane will most likely benefit from an interdisciplinary management with internist, pain specialist, psychiatrist, and/or psychologist working as a team. Integrative medicine approaches can also be offered in addition to her other treatment options, such as supplements (enzyme CoQ10, magnesium, butterbur) and energy healing to target the muscle memory from her car accident.

CONCLUSION

Careful history and examination are essential; further work-up such as a diagnostic blockade may be required, as the differential diagnosis and potential causes of cervicogenic headache are broad.

KEY POINTS TO REMEMBER

- Careful history and exam to evaluate for potential secondary causes such an arterial dissection, a posterior cranial fossa lesion, meningitis.
- By definition, cervicogenic headache is not due to cervical myofascial trigger points or cervical radiculopathy.
- If there are no red flags and the examination is unremarkable, a good first step for the management of neck pain/tension radiating to the head is physical therapy with or without low-dose tizanidine or trigger point injections to help gain some range of motion before starting or while waiting for physical therapy.
- Headache resolution from a block to a cervical structure or its nerve supply has both diagnostic and prognostic value.
- Radiofrequency denervation is the standard treatment for facet joint pain.

Further Reading

1. Bogduk N, Govind J. "Cervicogenic headache: an assessment of the evidence on clinical diagnosis, invasive tests, and treatment." *Lancet Neurol.* 2009;8(10):959–968. https://doi.org/10.1016/S1474-4422(09)70209-1.

2. Gehret J, Yadla S, Ratliff JK, Mandel S. "Evaluation of cervicalgia with headache." *Pract Neurol.* 2010; available at https://practicalneurology.com/articles/2010-nov-dec/evaluation-of-cervicalgia-with-headache.

3. Antonaci F, Fredriksen TA, Sjaastad O. "Cervicogenic headache: clinical presentation, diagnostic criteria, and differential diagnosis." *Curr Pain Headache Rep.* 2001;5(4):387–392. https://doi.org/10.1007/s11916-001-0030-1

4. Stovner LJ, Kolstad F, Helde G. "Radiofrequency denervation of facet joints C2–C6 in cervicogenic headache: a randomized, double-blind, sham-controlled study." *Cephalalgia.* 2004;24:821–830.

5. Lord SM, Barnsley L, Wallis BJ, McDonald GJ, Bogduk N. "Percutaneous radio-frequency neurotomy for chronic cervical zygapophyseal-joint pain." *N Engl J Med.* 1996;335:1721–1726.
6. Husted DS, Orton D, Schofferman J, Kine G. "Effectiveness of repeated radiofrequency neurotomy for cervical facet joint pain." *J Spinal Disord Tech.* 2008;21:406–408.
7. Hurley RW, Adams CB, Barad M, et al. "Consensus practice guidelines on interventions for cervical spine (facet) joint pain from a multispecialty international working group." *Pain Med.* 2021;22(11):2443–2524.

30 A New Headache Worse at Night and When Bending Down

Claire E. J. Ceriani and Hsiangkuo Yuan

Bernard is a 28-year-old man who comes to the office with a new persistent headache for 2 weeks. He has a history of occasional headaches he calls "sinus headaches" and describes as a throbbing pain behind his eyes accompanied by a clear nasal discharge, nausea, and photophobia. His usual headaches resolve with naproxen or acetaminophen. However, his current headache feels different from his prior headaches and improves minimally with medications. He describes a dull, achy feeling on the top of his head that worsens when he bends over. He does not have any facial pain or nasal discharge, but says his nose feels "blocked." The pain sometimes wakes him from sleep. A careful cranial nerve examination including fundoscopic exam and neurological exam are unremarkable.

What do I do now?

Diagnosis

Bernard gives a history of two different types of headaches. His long-standing occasional headaches that he self-diagnosed "sinus headaches" have some migraine features (throbbing pain, photophobia, nausea). Migraine may present with retro-orbital or facial pain, and activation of parasympathetic nerve fibers may cause autonomic symptoms such as rhinorrhea, which may lead to diagnostic confusion. Indeed, studies have evaluated patients with "sinus headaches" and found that 75%–90% met criteria for migraine or probable migraine. This patient most likely has a history of undiagnosed migraine.

His new headache, refractory and that wakes him up from sleep, warrants work-up with imaging. An MRI of the brain and sinuses is obtained, which shows fluid filling the bilateral sphenoid sinuses and the posterior right ethmoid air cells (see Figure 30.1). His MRI is concerning for acute bilateral sphenoid and right ethmoid rhinosinusitis.

A distinction between acute rhinosinusitis (ARS) and chronic rhinosinusitis (CRS) is usually made based on symptom duration, though CRS can sometimes cause bone sclerosis and demineralization that may be visible on imaging. According to the American Academy of Otolaryngology—Head and Neck Surgery (AAO-HNS) guidelines, rhinosinusitis with a duration of less than 4 weeks is ARS. A duration longer than 12 weeks would be diagnosed as CRS, and duration of 4 to 12 weeks may be termed subacute rhinosinusitis, though the AAO-HNS does not distinguish this as an explicit entity. CRS rarely causes headache and/or facial pain. A diagnosis of ARS is difficult to make, as there is a wide range of presentations that may not be captured by published diagnostic criteria. In cases like this, it is important to include sinus disease in the differential in patients presenting with atypical or new type of headache, and look at the sinuses when reviewing the brain imaging.

According to the International Classification of Headache Disorders 3rd Edition (ICHD-3) definition of 11.5.1 Headache attributed to acute rhinosinusitis, any headache phenotype is allowed, but there must be clinical, nasal endoscopic, or imaging evidence of ARS, as well as evidence of causation. Causation is demonstrated by two of the following: temporal relation, worsening or improvement of the headache and rhinosinusitis in parallel, exacerbation by pressure over the sinuses, and headache localized

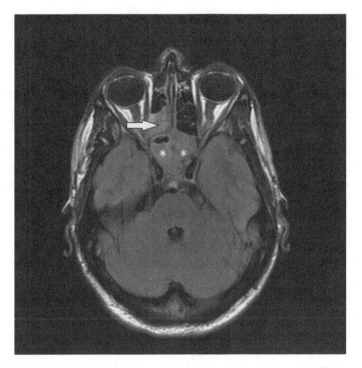

FIGURE 30.1 MRI showing fluid in the posterior right ethmoid air cells (arrow) and bilateral sphenoid sinuses (asterisks) with visible air-fluid level.

and ipsilateral to the site of rhinosinusitis if it is unilateral. Tenderness on palpation of the sinuses is not present in all patients, and headache location has not been shown to correlate with rhinosinusitis location on imaging, so these criteria may not be valid in all patients. Improvement of the headache and ARS in parallel can only be determined in retrospect. The criteria also do not specify what symptoms would constitute clinical evidence of ARS.

The most frequently described phenotype of headache attributed to ARS is like periorbital and frontal tension-type headache (pressure-like, dull, aching, or tightening). Other headache features include worsening with head movement (particularly bending forward), poor response to analgesics, interference with sleep, and nasal stuffiness or discharge. The pain location usually does not correlate with the location of rhinosinusitis on imaging. Migraine features such as nausea, photophobia, and phonophobia are present in a minority of patients.

The AAO-HNS guidelines define rhinosinusitis as purulent nasal discharge accompanied by nasal obstruction and/or facial pain-pressure-fullness. The differential diagnosis for facial pain is broad, and the inclusion of purulent nasal discharge in the diagnostic criteria increases the specificity for bacterial ARS. This reduces the likelihood of a patient with facial pain due to a primary headache disorder being misdiagnosed with rhinosinusitis, but it may miss a diagnosis of sphenoid rhinosinusitis, which may not present with purulent drainage until obstruction is relieved by surgery. Bernard has a history of clear nasal discharge with his previous headaches, but none with his current headache. His clear rhinorrhea would not meet criteria for rhinosinusitis, but neither does his current headache with no discharge at all.

The International Forum of Allergy and Rhinology (IFAR) guidelines allow for either nasal obstruction or nasal discharge accompanied by facial pain/pressure or reduction/loss of smell. These guidelines may capture patients without nasal discharge, but both the AAO-HNS and IFAR guidelines fail to capture rhinosinusitis in patients with head pain located somewhere other than the face, such as in this patient who has vertex pain.

A Diagnosis Not to Miss – Sphenoid Rhinosinusitis

Sphenoid rhinosinusitis deserves special consideration due to the difficulty of diagnosis and high rate of serious complications including meningitis, cavernous sinus thrombosis, abscess, hypophysitis, and ophthalmic disease. Sphenoid rhinosinusitis is most often associated with frontal or vertex pain, but pain can be anywhere in the head or face. It can sometimes present as thunderclap headache or have migrainous features with nausea and vomiting. It is usually worsened by bending, standing, and walking. It may be associated with fever and anosmia. Some patients may have visual symptoms, facial paresthesias, or other cranial nerve palsies. There may or may not be purulent discharge, and diagnostic nasal endoscopy may be negative. There is no single clinical feature with both high sensitivity and specificity for sphenoid rhinosinusitis, but experts recommend the diagnosis be considered in anyone with atypical headache that interferes with sleep, does not respond to simple analgesics, is exacerbated by head movement, or is accompanied by cranial nerve abnormalities. Neuroimaging is necessary for definitive diagnosis. Both CT and MRI may be used, but CT is generally preferred due to its cost effectiveness and better visualization of bone. If CT shows osseous destruction, extra-sinus extension, or local invasion, MRI should be obtained.

Differential Diagnosis

Other abnormalities of the sinuses that may present with headache include osteomas, fibrous dysplasia of the sinuses, tumors, and cerebral arachnoid cysts at the skull base. Septal deformations with a contact point on the lateral nasal wall can cause headache and are often missed on neuroimaging. Pain relief with local application of lidocaine predicts improvement with surgery. Contact points may also be seen on imaging in asymptomatic individuals, so their clinical significance is debated.

Treatment

Treatment of the underlying rhinosinusitis is necessary to treat the headache. Viral infections require only symptomatic care with simple analgesics, topical intranasal steroids, and/or nasal saline irrigation. Viral ARS symptoms usually peak within 3 days and resolve within 10 to 14 days. When symptoms last longer than 10 days, bacterial ARS should be suspected. Amoxicillin is first-line therapy, but this should be broadened to amoxicillin with clavulanate in patients with frontal or sphenoid ARS, and in those who are at risk of being infected with an amoxicillin-resistant organism (protracted symptoms, smoker, recent antibiotic use, working/living in a healthcare environment, immunocompromised). Because of the high rate of complications, patients with sphenoid involvement who are not improving after 24 hours of antibiotic treatment should be considered for urgent endoscopic sinus surgery.

KEY POINTS TO REMEMBER

- Headaches attributed to rhinosinusitis and primary headache disorders have overlapping symptoms that can complicate diagnosis.
- So-called "sinus headaches" are often migraine.

- Sinus disease should be in the differential for any patient with atypical headache, new type of headache, and/or nasal symptoms.
- Sphenoid rhinosinusitis has a high rate of complication but is easily missed due to lack of typical nasal symptoms.
- Headache attributed to rhinosinusitis should resolve once the infection has resolved. Patients with sphenoid involvement should be considered for urgent endoscopic sinus surgery.

Further Reading

1. Godley FA, Casiano RR, Mehle M, McGeeney B, Gottschalk C. "Update on the diagnostic considerations for neurogenic nasal and sinus symptoms: A current review suggests adding a possible diagnosis of migraine." *Am J Otolaryngol.* 2019;40(2):306–311.
2. Ceriani CEJ, Silberstein SD. "Headache and rhinosinusitis: a review." *Cephalalgia.* 2021;41(4):453–463.
3. Brooks I, Gooch WM, Jenkins SG, et al. "Medical management of acute bacterial sinusitis: Recommendations of a clinical advisory committee on pediatric and adult sinusitis." *Ann Otol Rhinol Laryngol Suppl.* 2000;182:2–20.
4. Tarabichi M. "Characteristics of sinus-related pain." *Otolaryngol Head Neck Surg.* 2000;122(6):842–847.
5. Rosenfeld RM, Piccirillo JF, Chandrasekhar SS, et al. "Clinical practice guideline (update): adult sinusitis." *Otolaryngol Head Neck Surg.* 2015;152(2 Suppl):S1–S39.
6. Deans JAJ, Welch AR. "Acute isolated sphenoid sinusitis: a disease with complications." *J Laryngol Otol.* 1991;105(12):1072–1074.
7. Ruoppi P, Seppa J, Pukkila M, Nuutinen J. "Isolated sphenoid sinus diseases: report of 39 cases." *Arch Otolaryngol Head Neck Surg.* 2000;126(6):777–781.
8. Charakorn N, Snidvongs K. "Chronic sphenoid rhinosinusitis: management challenge." *J Asthma Allergy.* 2016;9:199–205.
9. Farmer RL, Garg RK, Afifi AM. "Can functional nasal surgery treat chronic headaches? A systematic review." *Plast Reconstr Surg.* 2018;142(6):1583–1592.
10. Herzallah IR, Hamed MA, Salem SM, Suurna MV. "Mucosal contact points and paranasal sinus pneumatization: Does radiology predict headache causality?" *Laryngoscope.* 2015;125(9):2021–2026.

31 Shooting Pains Behind the Head

Victor C. Wang

A 25-year-old woman presents with periodic sharp pains that start at the back of the head and radiate forward to the top of the head, and sometimes to the forehead. The pain is usually on the right side, but she also sometimes experiences pain on the left side in the same distribution. She has been diagnosed in the past with migraine but does not experience any nausea, vomiting, or photophobia with the current pain. Sometimes the pain is felt behind the right eye. Magnetic resonance imaging (MRI) and magnetic resonance angiography (MRA) are unremarkable. She says that ibuprofen can sometimes decrease the pain. On exam, there is tenderness at the base of the skull on the right side with reproduction of her usual pain.

What do I do now?

Diagnosis

She has occipital neuralgia. Occipital neuralgia can sometimes be difficult to diagnose, as it can mimic other headache types, often from a unilateral pattern of pain. However, pain can sometimes be bilateral as well. Anatomically, the greater and lesser occipital nerves arise from the high cervical region to provide sensory innervation of the scalp. The patient will usually describe pain, tingling, shooting, burning, or other paresthesias in the distribution of the greater and/or lesser occipital nerve, starting at the top of the neck and radiating over the scalp to the top of the forehead (greater occipital nerve) and/or over the ear (lesser occipital nerve). The pain may reach the fronto-orbital area through trigeminocervical interneuronal connections in the trigeminal spinal nuclei. Sometimes the pain can be triggered over this distribution by touch, and a patient can report difficulty laying their head on a pillow. Patients will usually describe tenderness at the base of the skull, the back of the head, or the upper part of the neck.

The International Classification of Headache Disorders 3rd edition criteria for occipital neuralgia include unilateral or bilateral pain over the distribution of the greater and/or lesser occipital nerves, with at least two of these three characteristics: recurring in paroxysmal attacks lasting from a few seconds to minutes; severe intensity; and quality described as shooting, stabbing, or sharp. The pain is associated with dysesthesia and/or allodynia during stimulation of the scalp and/or hair, with tenderness over the nerve branches or trigger points at the emergence of the greater occipital nerve or in the distribution of the C2 dermatome. Finally, pain is improved with local diagnostic anesthetic.

Work-up

Diagnosis of occipital neuralgia is based primarily on history and exam, and a local nerve block can be performed to serve as an aid in diagnosis and treatment. Although most cases are idiopathic, MRI can be helpful in the rare cases of occipital neuralgia secondary to an impingement of the greater or lesser occipital nerves anywhere along the distribution of the nerve. Differential diagnosis for pain in the occipital region would include cervicogenic headache originating from the atlantoaxial or upper zygapophyseal joints, myofascial pain from cervical trigger points, migraine headache, and cluster headache.

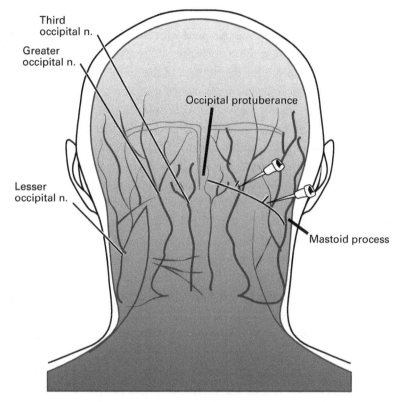

FIGURE 31.1 Anatomy for performing the greater occipital nerve and lesser occipital nerve block.

Treatment

Treatments of occipital neuralgia vary by provider, but medications and nerve blocks are often the initial form of treatment once diagnosis has been made. For medication therapy, four broad general classes of medications are used, which include anticonvulsants such as gabapentin or pregabalin, antidepressants such as tricyclics, NSAIDs, and/or muscle relaxants. Percutaneous nerve blocks are generally reserved for patients with more intractable symptoms.

There is no standardized technique for performing the occipital nerve block (see Figure 31.1. Most providers start by palpating the occipital protuberance as a starting landmark and then drawing a line to the mastoid process. The greater occipital nerve should lie about one-third the distance to the mastoid. The skin is then prepped with alcohol, and an injection of local anesthetic with or without corticosteroid is given. Patients will generally report numbness in the distribution of the nerve, and diagnostic improvement of pain as well. There are various techniques, but the American Headache Society published an expert consensus recommendation in 2013 describing the injection (see Blumenfeld et al. in Further Reading), using a 3–5 mL syringe and 25- to 30- gauge 0.5- to 1-inch needle inserted 3–4 mm. After negative aspiration to check that the needle is not intravascular, the injectate can be delivered either in one place or fanned. Injectate solution also varies by provider, but AHS recommendations describe lidocaine 1%–2% or bupivacaine 0.25%–5% with a volume of 1.5–3 mL per nerve. The lesser occipital nerve should run about two-thirds of the way from the same line between the occipital protuberance to the mastoid process. Using the same technique, 1–2 mL is the recommended injection per nerve. Peripheral nerve blocks with lidocaine are considered safe to perform during pregnancy. Corticosteroids such as triamcinolone, dexamethasone, methylprednisolone, or betamethasone are often mixed with the injectate solution to increase the duration of effect, though some providers elect to forgo steroid use altogether. Corticosteroid dosing is variable depending on provider preference. The major risks of corticosteroids are cutaneous atrophy and alopecia.

For intractable cases of occipital neuralgia, other experimental procedures have been tried including radiofrequency ablation of the nerve and botulinum toxin injections. Experimental surgical procedures such as peripheral nerve stimulation, spinal cord stimulation, and C2/C3 ganglionectomy have been performed with some success. Drawbacks of these procedures include permanent scalp numbness and possible return of symptoms over time.

KEY POINTS TO REMEMBER

- Occipital neuralgia can reach the fronto-orbital area.
- Occipital nerve blocks help to confirm the diagnosis and management.

- Treatment approach may be multimodal, with occipital nerve block, short course of NSAIDs, neck physical therapy, and preventive medications such as low-dose amitriptyline, for example.

Further Reading

1. Blumenfeld A, et al. "Expert consensus recommendations for the performance of peripheral nerve blocks for headaches—a narrative review." *Headache*. 2013;53(3):437–446. doi:10.1111/head.12053
2. Tobin J, Flitman S. "Occipital nerve blocks: When and what to inject?" *Headache*. 2009;49(10):1521–1533. https://doi.org/10.1111/j.1526-4610.2009.01493.x

Index

CT. *See* computed tomography
Cures Act, 9
CVST (cerebral venous sinus thrombosis), 104, 111, 123, 124

decision-making, xi, 14
depression
    cluster headache, 38
    giant cell arteritis, 119
    medication overuse/adaptation headache, 165
    new daily persistent headache, 65–66
    post-craniotomy headache, 99
    post-ischemic stroke headache, 105, 106
    screening for, 72*t*
diaries and calendars, 5, 12, 18, 29, 165
differential diagnosis, 3
ditans. *See also names of specific ditans*
    chronic migraine, 30–31
    migraine in pregnancy, 23–24

EBP (epidural blood patching), 24, 144–45, 146–48, 147*f*
EMDR (Eye Movement Desensitization and Reprocessing), 19
epidural blood patching (EBP), 24, 144–45, 146–48, 147*f*
estrogen
    menstrual migraine, 5
    migraine aura, 44
exercise, 12–14
    anxiety-triggered headache, 19
    cervicogenic headache, 175
    medication overuse/adaptation headache, 165
    migraine in pregnancy, 24
    reversible cerebral vasoconstriction syndrome, 126
    temporomandibular disorders, 72–73
Eye Movement Desensitization and Reprocessing (EMDR), 19

Feldenkreis work, 12–14

GCA. *See* giant cell arteritis
gepants. *See also names of specific gepants*
    chronic migraine, 30–31
    COVID-19-related headache, 171
    migraine in pregnancy, 23–24
    post-ischemic stroke headache, 105–6
giant cell arteritis (GCA), 115–20
    defined, 116
    diagnosis, 117–19
    differentiating from hypnic headache, 60
    differentiating from primary stabbing headache, 55
    differentiating from temporomandibular disorders, 71
    differentiating from trigeminal neuralgia, 86
    patterns of headache, 116
    spectrum of, 116
    symptoms of, 116–17
    treatment for, 119–20
    trigger for evaluation, 4
    work-up, 117–19

HaNDL (syndrome of transient headache and neurological deficits with cerebrospinal fluid lymphocytosis), 43
headache evaluation
    challenges of, xi, 2
    clinical history, xi, 2–3
    differential between new and different, 2–3
    flags, 3–5
    listening, xi, 2
    neurological examinations, xi, 3
    pain and symptom management, 5
hemicrania continua, 47–52
    diagnosis, 49–50
    differentiating from new daily persistent headache, 64
    prevalence of, 51
    treatment for, 49–50
    work-up, 48–49
herbs and vitamins, 12–14
hormonal replacement therapy, 44

Horner's syndrome, 76, 103–4
hypnic headache, 59–61
    diagnosis, 60
    treatment for, 60
    work-up, 60

ice-pick headache. *See* thunderclap headache
ICH. *See* intracerebral hemorrhage
idiopathic intracranial hypertension
        (IIH), 135–41
    children and, 139–40
    defined, 136
    diagnosis, 136
    pregnancy and, 139
    prognosis, 138
    symptoms of, 136
    treatment for, 137–38
    work-up, 136–37, 137*f*
indomethacin
    hemicrania continua, 49, 50–51
    hypnic headache, 60
    new daily persistent headache, 64
    primary stabbing headache, 56–57
integrative nutrition, 13*t*, 14
intracerebral hemorrhage (ICH)
    differentiating from cerebral amyloid
        angiopathy, 130, 131
    differentiating from thunderclap
        headache, 123–24
intracranial neoplasia, 60
ischemic stroke. *See* post-ischemic stroke
    headache

ketamine
    cluster headache, 38
    new daily persistent headache, 66–67

lactation and breastfeeding, 24–25
lamotrigine
    migraine aura, 43–44
    trigeminal neuralgia, 88*t*
lasmiditan
    chronic migraine, 30–31
    post-ischemic stroke headache, 105, 106

lithium
    cluster headache, 38
    hypnic headache, 60
loteprednol, 77–78
lumbar puncture, 3–4
    chronic migraine, 29–30
    COVID-19-related headache, 170
    idiopathic intracranal hypertension,
        137, 139–40
    new daily persistent headache, 65
    thunderclap headache, 123–24

magnesium, 94–95
magnetic resonance angiography (MRA)
    cerebral amyloid angiopathy, 130
    cluster headache, 37
    giant cell arteritis, 117–18
    hemicrania continua, 48–49
    new daily persistent headache, 65
    PCoA, 111
    post-ischemic stroke headache, 104
    primary stabbing headache, 55
    thunderclap headache, 124, 125*f*, 125
magnetic resonance imaging (MRI)
    acute rhinosinusitis-related headache,
        180, 181*f*
    brain neoplasm/tumor, 153
    cerebral amyloid angiopathy, 130, 131
    cerebrospinal fluid leak, 145–46
    cervicogenic headache, 175
    chronic migraine, 29–30
    cluster headache, 37
    giant cell arteritis, 117–18
    hemicrania continua, 48–49
    hypnic headache, 60
    idiopathic intracranial hypertension,
        136, 137*f*, 139
    incidental findings, 18
    new daily persistent headache, 65
    occipital neuralgia, 186
    PCoA, 111
    pituitary lesions, 158–60
    post-ischemic stroke headache,
        104, 105*f*

MRV. *See* magnetic resonance venography
multimodal approaches, xi

tension-type headache, 29, 54, 64, 94, 103, 116, 152, 164, 165, 174, 181
thunderclap headache (TCH), 121–27
  cervical artery dissection, 103–4
  diagnosis, 123
  differential diagnosis, 123
  differentiating from primary stabbing headache, 54
  management of, 126
  prognosis, 126–27
  red flags, 123
  vascular etiologies, 111
  work-up, 123–25
TMDs. *See* temporomandibular disorders
TN. *See* trigeminal neuralgia
tocilizumab (TCZ), 119–20
touch therapies, 12–14
transcutaneous supraorbital nerve stimulators, 32
traumatic head injury, 91–96
trigeminal autonomic cephalalgia (TAC), 47–52
  diagnosis, 49–50
  hemicrania continua, 48–49, 50
  prevalence of, 51
  treatment for, 49–50
  work-up, 48–49
trigeminal nerve
  anatomy of, 48*f*
  branches of, 84*t*
  compression of, 85–86
  corneal neuropathic pain, 78
  trigeminal autonomic cephalalgia, 49
  trigeminal neuralgia, 83–89
  visualization of, 85–86, 87*f*

trigeminal neuralgia (TN), 83–89
  classifications of, 85–86
  defined, 84
  diagnosis, 84–86
  red flags, 84–85, 85*t*
  treatment for, 86–89, 88*t*
  work-up, 86, 87*f*
triptans. *See also names of specific triptans*
  brain neoplasm/tumor-related headache, 153–54
  chronic migraine, 30–31
  COVID-19-related headache, 171
  medication overuse/adaptation headache, 164, 165–66
  migraine aura, 43, 44
  PCoA, 112
  post-ischemic stroke headache, 105

ubrogepant, 30–31
ultrasonography
  giant cell arteritis, 55, 117–18, 119
  red flags warranting, 4

V1. *See* ophthalmic division
V2. *See* maxillary division
V3. *See* mandibular division
visual aura rating scale, 5
visual therapies, 95
vitamin D, 38, 119
VNS (vagal nerve stimulator) devices, 32, 171–72

yoga, 12–14, 144

zolmitriptan, 30